Rethinking the *Brain*

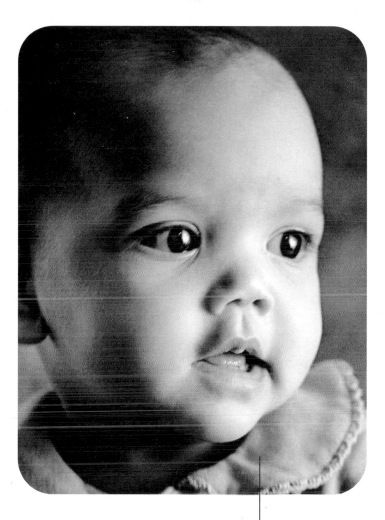

New Insights
into Early
Development

By Rima Shore

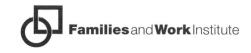

Families and **Work** Institute

ISBN 1-888324-04-X

Rethinking the Brain: New Insights into Early Development

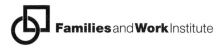 **Families** and **Work** Institute

Families and Work Institute is a non-profit organization that addresses the changing nature of work and family life. The Institute is committed to finding research-based strategies that foster mutually supportive connections among workplaces, families, and communities.

Some other Families and Work Institute publications:

Rethinking The Brain: Early Childhood Brain Development Presentation Kit

Community Mobilization: Strategies to Support Young Children and Their Families

Working Fathers: New Strategies for Balancing Work and Family

The 1997 National Study of the Changing Workforce

Ahead of the Curve: Why America's Leading Employers Are Addressing the Needs of New and Expectant Parents

New Expectations: Community Strategies for Responsible Fatherhood

The 1998 Business Work-Life Study: A Sourcebook

Families and Work Institute's

Corporate Leadership Circle

Corporate Benefactors
($15,000 or more)

AT&T

IBM Corporation

Johnson & Johnson

Joseph E. Seagram & Sons, Inc.

Merck & Co., Inc.

Pfizer Inc.

Corporate Patrons
($10,000–$14,999)

Aetna, Inc.

Bell Atlantic

Chase Manhattan Bank

Chevron Corporation

Eli Lilly and Company

General Electric Company

Marriott International

Prudential Insurance Company of America

Viacom, Inc.

Warner-Lambert Company

Xerox Corporation

Corporate Sponsors
($5,000–$9,999)

Allstate Insurance Company

Bright Horizons Family Solutions

Ceridian Corporation

Ernst & Young LLP

Fel-Pro Incorporated

Hallmark Cards, Inc.

PricewaterhouseCoopers

Sequent Computer Systems, Inc.

State Farm Insurance

Texas Instruments

WFD

Corporate Friends
($1,000–$4,999)

Baxter Healthcare Corporation

Burson-Marsteller

Champion International Corporation

Chubb Group of Insurance Companies

CIGNA Corporation

First Tennessee Bank

GTE

John Hancock Mutual Life Insurance Company

Hilton Hotels Corporation

Mutual of New York

Royal Bank of Canada

The Equitable Life Assurance Society

Time Warner, Inc.

Our thanks to these companies for annual donations for general operating support of the Institute.

Brain Development in Young Children

New Frontiers for Research, Policy, and Practice

Conference Funders

Carnegie Corporation of New York

The Harris Foundation

The Charles A. Dana Foundation

McCormick Tribune Foundation

Conference Steering Committee

Duane Alexander, MD
Director
National Institute of Child Health
and Human Development

Heidelise Als, PhD
Associate Professor of Psychology
Harvard Medical School

Denise Carter Blank, PhD
Director of Education Programs
McCormick Tribune Foundation

Donald J. Cohen, MD
Professor and Director
Yale Child Study Center

Felton Earls, MD
Professor of Human Behavior
Harvard School of Public Health

Emily Fenichel, MSW
Associate Director
ZERO TO THREE

Ellen Galinsky, MS
President
Families and Work Institute

Irving B. Harris
Chairman
The Harris Foundation

Michael H. Levine, PhD
Program Officer
Carnegie Corporation of New York

Margaret E. Mahoney
President
MEM Associates, Inc.

Jim O'Sullivan
Program Officer
The Charles A. Dana Foundation

Deborah Phillips, PhD
Director
Board on Children and Families of
the National Research Council

Barry Zuckerman, MD
Chief and Chairman, Department
of Pediatrics
Boston University Medical School

Funders of the "I Am Your Child" Early Childhood Public Engagement Campaign

The conference from which this publication springs was one of the first steps in the "I Am Your Child" campaign, a national public awareness and engagement campaign to make early childhood development a priority for our nation. Campaign founders include Rob Reiner, Michele Singer Reiner, and Ellen Gilbert of International Creative Management, as well as a broad range of experts from the early childhood fields. The Families and Work Institute is coordinating outreach activities for this effort. The campaign is made possible through the generous support of the following foundations and corporate sponsors:

AT&T Foundation

The California Wellness
Foundation

Carnegie Corporation of New York

The Commonwealth Fund

The Charles A. Dana
Foundation, Inc.

Freddie Mac Foundation

The Harris Foundation

The Teresa & H. John Heinz III
Foundation

IBM Corporation

Johnson & Johnson

W.K. Kellogg Foundation

The Robert Wood Johnson
Foundation

John D. & Catherine T. MacArthur
Foundation

A.L. Mailman Family
Foundation, Inc.

McCormick Tribune Foundation

The Travelers Foundation

Funding for printing this publication was provided by the McCormick Tribune Foundation.

The following individuals donated their time and expertise to read—
and in some cases re-read—this publication in manuscript.

Larry Aber, PhD
Director
National Center for Children
in Poverty

April Ann Benasich, PhD
Assistant Professor of Neuroscience
and Director of Infancy Studies
Center for Molecular and Behavioral
Neuroscience
Rutgers University

James Black, MD, PhD
Assistant Professor of Psychiatry
University of Illinios
Urbana Champaign

Barbara T. Bowman, MA
President
Erikson Institute

Harry Chugani, MD
Director, PET Center
Professor of Pediatrics, Neurology and
Radiation
Director of Epilepsy
Surgery Program
Wayne State University
Medical School

Geraldine Dawson, PhD
Professor of Psychology
Department of Psychology
University of Washington

Felton Earls, MD
Professor of Human Behavior
and Development
Harvard School of Public Health

Martha Farrell Erickson, PhD
Director
Children Youth and Family Consortium
University of Minnesota

Emily Fenichel, MSW
Associate Director
ZERO TO THREE

James Garbarino, PhD
Director
Family Life Development Center
Cornell University

William T. Greenough, PhD
Professor of Psychology, Psychiatry
and Cell and Structural Biology
University of Illinois
Urbana Champaign

Stanley Greenspan, MD
Clinical Professor of Psychiatry,
Behavioral Sciences and Pediatrics
George Washington University
Medical Center

Megan Gunnar, PhD
Distinguished McNight University
Professor of Child Development
Institute of Child Development
University of Minnesota

Myron A. Hofer, PhD
Professor of Psychiatry
Director, Division of Developmental
Psychobiology
Columbia University College of
Physicians and Surgeons

Ronald Kotulak
Science Writer
Chicago Tribune

Ronald Lally, EdD
Director, Center for Child & Family
Studies
WESTED/Far West Laboratory

Judy Langford Carter
Former Executive Director
Family Resource Coalition

Bennett L. Levanthal, MD
Chairman (Interim)
Department of Psychiatry
Director of Child and Adolescent
Psychiatry
The University of Chicago

Margaret E. Mahoney
President
MEM Associates, Inc.

Linda C. Mayes, MD
Arnold Gesell Associate Professor of
Child Development
Pediatrics and Psychology
Yale University Child
Study Center

Tracy Orleans, PhD
Senior Research and Program Officer
The Robert Wood Johnson Foundation

Bruce D. Perry, MD, PhD
Director, Civitas Child Trauma
Programs
Baylor College of Medicine

Deborah Phillips, PhD
Director
Board on Children, Youth and
Families of the
National Research Council

Pasko Rakic, MD, ScD
Professor and Chairman
Section of Neurobiology
Yale University School of Medicine

L. Alan Sroufe, PhD
William Harris Professor of
Child Psychology
Institute of Child Development
University of Minnesota

Kathryn Taaffe Young, PhD
Assistant Vice President
The Commonwealth Fund

Lauren Wakschlag, PhD
Department of Psychiatry
University of Chicago

Bernice Weissbourd, MA
President
Family Focus

Edward Zigler, PhD
Sterling Professor of Psychology
Director of the Bush Center
Yale University

Barry Zuckerman, MD
Chief and Chairman, Department of
Pediatrics
Boston University Medical Center

Our thanks to the following **Families and Work Institute** staff who contributed to this publication:
Jennifer E. Swanberg, John Boose, Nik Elevitch, Robin Hardman, and Tory Haskell.
We are also grateful to Barbara Shore for editorial and research support.

Table of Contents

Where Do We Go *From Here?*

Glossary

Appendices

Notes

Sources for Sidebars

Bibliography

Executive Summary

A father comforts a crying newborn. A mother plays peekaboo with her ten-month-old. A child care provider reads to a toddler. And in a matter of seconds, thousands of cells in these children's growing brains respond. Some brain cells are "turned on," triggered by this particular experience. Many existing connections among brain cells are strengthened. At the same time, new connections are formed, adding a bit more definition and complexity to the intricate circuitry that will remain largely in place for the rest of these children's lives.

We didn't always know it worked this way. Until recently, it was not widely believed that the brains of human infants could be so active and so complex. Nor did we realize how flexible the brain is. Only 15 years ago, neuroscientists assumed that by the time babies are born, the structure of their brains is genetically determined. They did not recognize that the experiences that fill a baby's first days, months and years have such a decisive impact on the architecture of their brains, or on the nature and extent of their adult capacities. Today, thanks in part to decades of research on brain chemistry and sophisticated new technologies, neuroscientists are providing evidence for assertions that would have been greeted with skepticism ten or twenty years ago.

Breakthroughs in Neuroscience—Why Now?

Every field of endeavor has peak moments of discovery and opportunity, when past knowledge converges with new needs, new insights, and new technologies to produce stunning advances. For neuroscience, this is one such moment. Certainly, the development of new research tools, such as brain imaging technologies, has been a crucial factor. But technological advances never occur in a vacuum. Brain research has been stimulated, in part, by growing concern about the status of children in America—not only their academic achievement, but also their health, safety, and overall well-being. There is growing consensus, among decision makers in many fields, that efforts to recast policy and reconsider the best use of public resources must begin at the beginning—with clearheaded thinking about young children's brains.

What Have We Learned?

1. **Human development hinges on the interplay between nature and nurture.** Much of our thinking about the brain has been dominated by old assumptions— that the genes we are born with determine how our brains develop, and that in turn how our brains develop determines how we interact with the world. Recent brain research challenges these assumptions. Neuroscientists have found that throughout the entire process of development, beginning even before birth, the brain is affected by environmental conditions, including the kind of nourishment, care, surroundings, and stimulation an individual receives. The impact of the environment is dramatic and specific, not merely influencing the general direction of development, but actually affecting how the intricate circuitry of the brain is wired.

The notion of "wiring" or "circuitry" is often used to describe the brain's complex network. Brain function hinges on the rapid, efficient passage of signals from one part of the brain to another. It needs a well organized network. The building blocks of this network are brain cells (neurons) and the connections (synapses) they form to other brain cells. These synapses are vital to healthy development and learning: they link up to form neural pathways. As an individual interacts with the environment—reacting to stimuli, taking in information, processing it, or storing it—new signals race along these neural pathways. In neuroscientists' terms, the synapses and the pathways they form are "activated."

It is during the first three years of life that the vast majority of synapses is produced. The number of synapses increases with astonishing rapidity until about age three and then holds steady throughout the first decade of life. A child's brain becomes super-dense, with twice as many synapses as it will eventually need. Brain development is, then, a process of pruning.

This is why early experience is so crucial: those synapses that have been activated many times by virtue of repeated early experience tend to become permanent; the synapses that are not used often enough tend to be eliminated. In this way early experiences—positive or negative—have a decisive impact on how the brain is wired.

New knowledge about brain function should end the "nature or nurture" debate once and for all. A great deal of new research leads to this conclusion: how humans develop and learn depends critically and continually on the interplay between nature (an individual's genetic endowment) and nurture (the nutrition, surroundings, care, stimulation, and teaching that are provided or withheld). Both are crucial.

2. | Early care has a decisive and long-lasting impact on how people develop, their ability to learn, and their capacity to regulate their own emotions. The ways that parents, families, and other caregivers relate and respond to young children, and the ways that they mediate children's contact with the environment, directly affect the formation of neural pathways. In particular, a child's capacity to control emotions appears to hinge, to a significant extent, on biological systems shaped by his or her early experiences and attachments. Neuroscientists are finding that a strong, secure attachment to a nurturing caregiver can have a protective biological function, helping a growing child withstand (and, indeed, learn from) the ordinary stresses of daily life. There is no single "right" way to create this capacity; warm, responsive care can take many forms.

3. | The human brain has a remarkable capacity to change, but timing is crucial. There is mounting evidence that the brain has the capacity to change in important ways in response to experience. It shows that the brain is not a static entity, and that an individual's capacities are not fixed at birth. The brain itself can be altered—or helped to compensate for problems—with timely, intensive intervention. In the first decade of life, and particularly in the first few years, the brain's ability to change and compensate is especially remarkable.

Because the brain has the capacity to change, there are ample opportunities to promote and support children's healthy growth and development. But timing is crucial. While learning continues throughout the life cycle, there are optimal periods of opportunity—"prime times"—during which the brain is particularly efficient at specific types of learning. In the neurobiological literature, these times are called "critical periods."

4. **There are times when negative experiences or the absence of appropriate stimulation are more likely to have serious and sustained effects.** A number of researchers have focused their attention on specific circumstances that may interfere with warm, responsive caregiving during critical periods, including maternal depression. While not all babies of depressed mothers show negative effects, maternal depression can impede healthy brain development, particularly in the part of the brain associated with the expression and regulation of emotions. Postpartum depression that lasts only a few months does not appear to have a lasting impact; but babies who are from six to eighteen months old when their mothers suffer from depression appear to be at greater risk. When mothers are treated for or recover from depression, their children's brain activity and behavior can improve significantly.

New knowledge about the vulnerability of the developing brain to environmental factors suggests that significant, early exposure to such substances as nicotine, alcohol, and cocaine may have more harmful and long-lasting effects on young children than was previously suspected.

Early experiences of trauma or ongoing abuse, whether in utero or after birth, can interfere with the development of the subcortical and limbic areas of the brain, resulting in extreme anxiety, depression, and/or the inability to form healthy attachments to others. Adverse experiences throughout childhood can also impair cognitive abilities.

Many of the risk factors described above occur together, jeopardizing the healthy development of young children and making research endeavors more challenging. Research shows that many of these risk factors are associated with or exacerbated by poverty. Today, fully a quarter of American children under the age of six are growing up in poverty; the same figure holds for children under the age of three. Economic deprivation affects their nutrition, access to medical care, the safety and predictability of their physical environment, the level of family stress, and the quality and continuity of their day-to-day care.

5. **Evidence amassed over the last decade points to the wisdom and efficacy of prevention and early intervention.** There are, to be sure, some genetic disorders or neurological events (such as a massive stroke) whose consequences are difficult if not impossible to reverse, given current knowledge and methods. But study after study shows that intensive, well designed, timely intervention can improve the prospects—and the quality of life—of many children who are considered to be at risk of cognitive, social, or emotional impairment. In some cases, effective intervention efforts can even ameliorate conditions once thought to be virtually untreatable, such as autism or mental retardation.

The efficacy of early intervention has been demonstrated and replicated in diverse communities across the nation. Children from families with the least formal education appear to derive the greatest cognitive benefits from intervention programs. Moreover, the impact of early intervention appears to be long-lasting, particularly when there is follow-up during the elementary school years.

Where Do We Go From Here?

In most spheres of knowledge, what we don't know far exceeds what we do know. Brain research is no exception. Coming years promise to yield new discoveries about how the brain develops and how children's capacities grow and mature.

However, the knowledge base is ample enough to allow us to act now. A framework for action might be designed around key assertions presented in this report, including the importance of the interplay between nature and nurture; the importance of strong, secure early attachments; the extent and rapidity of early development; the brain's remarkable plasticity; and the wisdom and efficacy of prevention and high-quality, well designed early intervention.

Such a framework would need to take into account three key principles:

First, do no harm. New insights into the brain suggest that the principle that guides medical practice should be applied just as rigorously to all policies and practices that affect children: first do no harm. Policies or practices that prevent parents from forming strong, secure attachments with their infants in the first months of life need urgent attention and reform. At the same time, parents need more information about how the kind of care they provide affects their children's capacities. "First, do no harm" also means mounting intensive efforts to improve the quality of child care and early education, so that parents can be sure that while they are at work, their young children's emotional development and learning are being fostered.

Prevention is best, but when a child needs help, intervene quickly and intensively. Knowing that early experience has such a strong influence on brain development, parents may worry that every unpleasant sensation or upsetting experience will become a neurological nightmare. They may rest assured that in most cases, a history of consistent and responsive care cushions children from the occasional bumps and bruises that are inevitable in everyday life. In most cases, children can recover even from serious stress or trauma. And if they are given timely, intensive, sustained help, they can overcome a wide range of developmental problems. More detailed knowledge about specific aspects of brain development and functioning will allow the design of interventions that more closely match children's needs.

Promote the healthy development and learning of every child. If we miss early opportunities to promote healthy development and learning, later remediation may be more difficult and expensive, and may be less effective given the knowledge, methods and settings that are currently available. However, *risk is not destiny*. The medical, psychological, and educational literatures contain sufficient examples of people who develop or recover significant capacities after critical periods have passed to sustain hope for every individual. Ongoing efforts to enhance the cognitive, emotional, and social development of youth and adults in every phase of the life cycle must be supported.

■ | Implications for Policy and Practice
New insights into early development confront policy makers and practitioners in many fields with thorny questions and difficult choices. As we move into the next century, our children need and deserve policies and practices that reflect the importance of the early years, and that embody the principles that emerged from the brain conference. In particular, new knowledge about early development adds weight and urgency to the following policy goals:

Improve health and protection by providing preventive and primary health care coverage for expectant and new parents and their young children. Today, about one in five pregnant women receives little or no prenatal care in the crucial first trimester; for African American, Latina, and American Indian women, the figure is one in three. In addition to prenatal care, pregnant women need safe homes, adequate nutrition, and buffering from extreme stress. The first three years of life are also filled with important health and safety risks, but millions of children in this age span are uninsured or underinsured.

Promote responsible parenthood by expanding proven approaches. All parents can benefit from solid information and support as they raise their children; some need more intensive assistance. There is substantial research evidence that certain parent education/family support programs promote the healthy development of children, improve the well-being of parents, and are cost-effective.

Safeguard children in child care from harm and promote their learning and development. Researchers have found that most child care settings are of mediocre to poor quality, and the nation's youngest children are the most likely to be in unsafe, substandard child care. More than one-third are in situations that can be detrimental to their development. Most of the rest are in settings where minimal learning is taking place. We can do better. Studies show that it is possible to improve quality, creating settings in which children can thrive and learn.

Enable communities to have the flexibility and the resources they need to mobilize on behalf of young children and their families. Efforts are now underway across the nation to mobilize communities on behalf of young children and their families. These efforts need and deserve support from national, state, and local leaders, as well as from leaders of business, the media, community organizations, and religious institutions.

■ Conveying New Knowledge about the Brain Finally, new knowledge about the brain must be communicated to families and the public at large with immense care. While mothers and fathers have a powerful impact on their children's development and learning, many factors play a role and parents must not be made to feel solely responsible for every hurdle their children may encounter. While warm, responsive caregiving helps to promote healthy development, some neurological conditions remain fairly resistant to change. And while the neuroscientist's lens may appear to magnify or isolate such neurological problems, they are in fact only one facet of these children's rich and complex lives.

The notion of critical periods also needs to be carefully qualified. To be sure, nature provides prime times for development and learning, but parents and other caregivers can take advantage of these times in many ways, drawing upon their own varied resources and beliefs. Moreover, it is never too late to improve the quality of a child's life.

In short, new insights into early brain development suggest that as we care for our youngest children, as we institute policies or practices that affect their day-to-day experience, the stakes are very high. But we can take comfort in the knowledge that there are many ways that we as parents, as caregivers, as citizens, and as policy makers can raise healthy, happy, smart children. We can take heart in the knowledge that there are many things that we as a nation can do, starting now, to brighten their future and ours.

Foreword

Rethinking the Brain, and the conference which inspired it, present an overview of neuroscientists' recent findings about the brain, and suggest how these insights can guide and support our nation's efforts to promote the healthy development and learning of young children.

What can science teach? How can its findings be applied to urgent social problems? Richard Feynman, a Nobel Laureate in physics, often mused about such questions. He wrote:

> *From time to time people suggest to me that scientists ought to give more consideration to social problems, especially that they should be more responsible in considering the impact of science on society. It seems to be generally believed that if the scientists would only look at these very difficult social problems and not spend so much time fooling with less vital scientific ones, great success would come of it. It seems to me that we do think about these problems, from time to time, but ... social problems are very much harder than scientific ones....*

Feynman went on to say that it would be a mistake to underestimate the value of the world view which comes from scientific endeavor. In particular, the wonders of science have led us "to imagine all sorts of things infinitely more marvelous than the imaginings of poets and dreamers of the past."

I have my own example of the wonders of imagination flowing from scientific findings. A human baby develops from the fertilization of a human egg by a human sperm, resulting in a combined cell which is very tiny. In about 25 weeks that microscopic cell grows to become a fetus weighing one pound. In 15 more weeks, the fetus grows sevenfold. I am awed by the fact that a fetus weighing one pound already has 100 billion brain cells (called neurons), any one of which may form, over time, as many as 15,000 connections to other brain cells.

This report is about the early development of the human brain. For many years, I have been interested in early childhood development. I have listened to and read the remarkable insights of people like Anna Freud, John Bowlby, the Robertsons of London, Selma Fraiberg, Berry Brazelton, and Sally Provence. I have been struck by the keen clinical judgments they reached about the importance of infancy, relying only on their own keen eyes, without the benefit of the new, sophisticated imaging technologies.

In the years when most of these pioneers began publishing their observations and theories, there was very little neurobiological evidence to confirm their judgments about the critical nature of early brain development. But over the last decade, incredible advances in the knowledge and tools available to neuroscientists have allowed them to document the immense proliferation of neurons in the prenatal period, as well as the processes by which children's brains, including those of infants, form myriad connections among those neurons. Indeed, how children's brains develop from a few cells to a complex structure encompassing billions of cells and trillions of connections is so astonishing as to be almost unbelievable.

Neuroscientists' insights suggest that the early years are filled with opportunities—and pitfalls. It is my hope that this report, and the discussions it sparks, will help parents, educators, human services providers, and policy makers in many fields seize those opportunities and sidestep those pitfalls.

Irving Harris
The Harris Foundation
April 1997

Preface

Rethinking the Brain is based, in large part, on the proceedings from a national conference that we organized and convened on the critical importance of early brain development for our nation's future well-being. This meeting, titled *Brain Development in Young Children: New Frontiers for Research, Policy and Practice*, was held on June 13 and 14, 1996 at the University of Chicago and brought together 150 of the nation's leading brain scientists, experts in child development and early education, business leaders, policy makers and members of the news media.

The conference has served as a research base for the "I Am Your Child" Campaign, an early childhood public engagement campaign established by Rob Reiner and Michele Singer Reiner; Ellen Gilbert of International Creative Management; and other prominent entertainers, media, foundations, corporations, and child development experts. The outreach campaign is coordinated by the Families and Work Institute. The campaign is bringing national attention to the importance of the first three years of life, promoting family involvement in young children's healthy development and school readiness, helping to mobilize communities to act on behalf of young children and their families, and building the capacity of early childhood organizations to help families nurture their children.

The conference on brain development and its report build on a seminal report, *Starting Points: Meeting the Needs of Our Youngest Children*, released by Carnegie Corporation of New York in 1994. *Starting Points* noted that:

> *Across the United States, we are beginning to hear the rumblings of a quiet crisis. Our nation's children under the age of three and their families are in trouble, and their plight worsens every day.*

> *To be sure, the children themselves are not quiet; they are crying out for help. And their parents' anxieties about inadequate child care and the high cost of their child's health care can be heard in kitchens, playgrounds, pediatricians' waiting rooms, and workplace cafeterias across the nation. But these sounds rarely become sound-bites.*

When *Starting Points* was released, much of the extensive media attention focused on new highly persuasive evidence from research on brain development that how individuals function from the preschool years all the way through adolescence and even adulthood hinges, to an important extent, on their experiences in the first three years of life.

But *Starting Points* also made it clear that there is a very wide gap between scientific research and public knowledge—between what is known and what is done. In particular, our nation's pivotal institutions have not carefully considered our growing knowledge of early brain development.

The conference amplified the information presented in *Starting Points*. This report began as a summary of information and perspectives presented at that conference. As it took shape, however, it grew into a more comprehensive effort to bring to public attention the following key findings of recent brain research:

- Human development hinges on the interplay between nature and nurture.
- Early care and nurture have a decisive and long-lasting impact on how people develop, their ability to learn, and their capacity to regulate their emotions.
- The human brain has a remarkable capacity to change, but timing is crucial.

- There are times when negative experiences or the absence of appropriate stimulation are more likely to have serious and sustained effects.
- Substantial evidence amassed by neuroscientists and child development experts over the last decade points to the wisdom and efficacy of prevention and early intervention.

These findings—as presented in *Rethinking the Brain*—are undergirded by substantial, hard scientific evidence collected painstakingly in research laboratories and through naturalistic observation. When considered together with the research of developmental psychologists and early intervention program experts, they expand the frontiers of knowledge; moreover, they should now compel public attention toward a much more forceful commitment to nurturing our youngest children.

This report is intended primarily for professionals in diverse fields who are seeking to achieve better results for young children and their families. We recognize, however, that the difficult choices it presents may raise concern for other members of the public, especially parents.

Rethinking the Brain highlights opportunities to promote healthy development, and to reduce risks, in the early years of life. In the process, it necessarily paints in broad strokes some very complex issues and debates. We wish to underscore that myriad factors shape a child's development—not only genes, but also the environment; and not only the immediate environment of the home, but also the larger social and economic settings of local communities and states, and of the nation as a whole. In this sense, all Americans share responsibility for every child.

Of course, parents bear the greatest responsibility for children's well-being. We believe that new insights into early development can help parents rethink their own approaches to childrearing and make sound decisions for their families. But no parent should draw from this report the conclusion that he or she is solely responsible for any difficulties a child may have.

As we rethink the brain, it is also vital to consider effective ways to present new findings to the public, with a view toward offering families help and hope, not distress or guilt. Research is needed to guide this effort. At the same time, we need the best thinking of leaders in diverse fields to address, on an ongoing basis, critical dissemination issues.

We are very grateful to the scholars and child development experts who participated in the conference and who reviewed this report; many spent hours with us, exploring the connections between the biological and the social sciences.

We were also especially fortunate to have a superb steering committee that helped shape the conference agenda and the subsequent report—led by the indefatigable and remarkable Irving Harris. His vision guided us through this entire process.

A special note of appreciation to Rima Shore. In addition to her lucid, artful prose and exceptional understanding of complex subjects, large and small, she has gone beyond the confines of the conference to incorporate additional research, presenting an in-depth picture of why and how we need to "rethink" the brain development of young children. We are also grateful to Jennifer Swanberg of the Families and Work Institute. She was an astute, tireless researcher while also managing the complex process of producing this report.

It is our strong hope that this report will make new insights into early development accessible to the public and policy makers, and that they will become the basis for taking action on behalf of young children and their families.

Ellen Galinsky
Families and Work Institute

Michael H. Levine
Carnegie Corporation of New York

April 1997

"*Beeboo*," she says.

"Peekaboo," her mother answers, spreading one hand in front of her face and trying to change her diaper with the other.

"Beebeebeebeebee," she sings, waving her arms excitedly.

"Peekaboo, I see you. There's my baby!"

And in a matter of seconds, thousands of cells in this child's growing brain respond. Some brain cells are "turned on," triggered by this particular experience. Many existing connections among brain cells are strengthened. At the same time, new connections are formed, adding a bit more definition and complexity to the intricate circuitry that will remain largely in place for the rest of her life.

We didn't always know it worked this way. Until recently, it was not widely believed that the brains of human infants could be so active and so complex. Nor did we realize how flexible the brain is. Only 15 years ago, neuroscientists assumed that by the time babies are born, the structure of their brains is genetically determined. They did not recognize that the experiences that fill a baby's first days, months, and years have such a decisive impact on the architecture of her brain, or on the nature and extent of her adult capacities. Nor did they appreciate the extent to which young children actively participate in their own brain development by signalling their needs to caregivers and by responding selectively to different kinds of stimulation.

Today, thanks in part to decades of research on brain chemistry and sophisticated new technologies, neuroscientists are providing evidence for assertions that would have been greeted with skepticism—if not outright disbelief—ten or twenty years ago. Of course, there is still some resistance to theories that challenge traditional ways of thinking about young children and about brain development. But now, teams of scientists across the nation and around the globe are elaborating on the brain's development and functions—getting right down to the cellular level. They are showing how nature and nurture interact on a continuous basis as children grow and mature. And in the process, they are sending a wake-up call to parents,

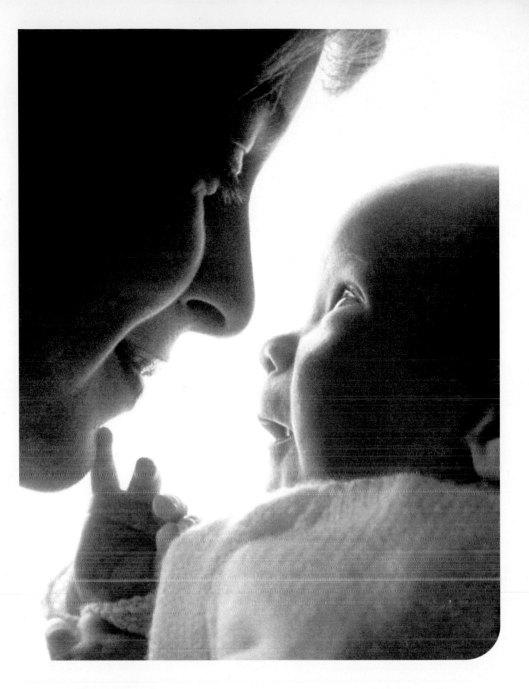

teachers, health professionals, and policy makers in many fields, cautioning that we ignore the opportunities and

risks of the first years of life at our own peril—and at the peril of future generations.

Indeed, brain research is one of the most exciting and fruitful scientific endeavors of the last decades of the

20th century. But unless this research finds its way into our homes and health clinics, our early childhood centers

and classrooms, America's schools and human service institutions will remain locked in a 19th-century paradigm.

"An Organ of Minor Importance"

How we function as adults hinges to a significant extent on how our brains develop when we are young. This statement may sound self-evident, but has not always held sway in public life. Indeed, resistance to brain research has a long and complex history that goes back to ancient times. Many people have resisted an emphasis on the brain because it seems to diminish the role of moral qualities, of "character" and "soul." In the fourth century B.C., Aristotle described the brain as "an organ of minor importance," insisting that "the seat of the soul and the control of voluntary movement—in fact, of nervous functions in general—are to be sought in the heart."

Few people today would endorse the notion that the brain has little importance, but many share the sense that the way to improve the status of America's children is to focus more on qualities of heart (the realm of families and clergy) than on the brain (the realm of scientists and academics). But in fact, by highlighting the interplay between nature and nurture, recent brain research challenges this dichotomy, stressing the vital role of families and communities in promoting optimal brain development.

Others have been wary of neuroscience because some of its early practitioners, including adherents of phrenology, used fallacious arguments about the brain to justify the subjugation of women, racial minorities, and immigrant groups. As a result of this ignoble history, many people understandably greet new efforts to lend scientific credibility to views about how and why people learn with some skepticism.

Finally, still others are reluctant today to lend credibility to brain research because they fear, with some reason, that it may be used to support a misinformed determinism—the conviction that young children have preset limits to what they can learn, or that we might as well give up on children who have not made a good start, academically, emotionally, or socially, in the first decade of life.

That is why it is so important to underscore three key findings of recent brain research:

- First, an individual's capacity to learn and thrive in a variety of settings depends on the interplay between nature (their genetic endowment) and nurture (the kind of care, stimulation, and teaching they receive).

- Second, the human brain—across all ethnic and racial groups—is uniquely constructed to benefit from experience and from good teaching, particularly during the first years of life.

- And third, while the opportunities and risks are greatest during the first years of life, learning takes place throughout the human life cycle.

In June 1996, a two-day conference was convened by the Families and Work Institute to discuss new knowledge about early brain development and its implications for America's children. Entitled *Brain Development in Young Children: New Frontiers for Research, Policy and Practice*, the conference was funded by the Carnegie Corporation of New York, The Charles A. Dana Foundation, The Harris Foundation and the McCormick Tribune Foundation, and was developed in conjunction with the "I Am Your Child" campaign, a public engagement effort designed to focus attention on the importance of the first three years of life.

The conference sprang from the conviction that not just parents and families, but the nation as a whole, has a vital stake in its youngest children's healthy development and learning. It brought together professionals from the neurosciences, medicine, education, human services, the media, business, and public policy to look at what is known about the brain and how that knowledge can and should inform efforts to improve results for children and their families.

This report draws on the proceedings of that conference as well as papers by participants, a range of other background materials and interviews with scholars. It highlights the major findings reported at the conference, summarizes their implications for policy and practice in education and the human services, notes areas of debate, and points to pathways for future research. Finally, it frames the tough policy questions that arise from new insights into early development.

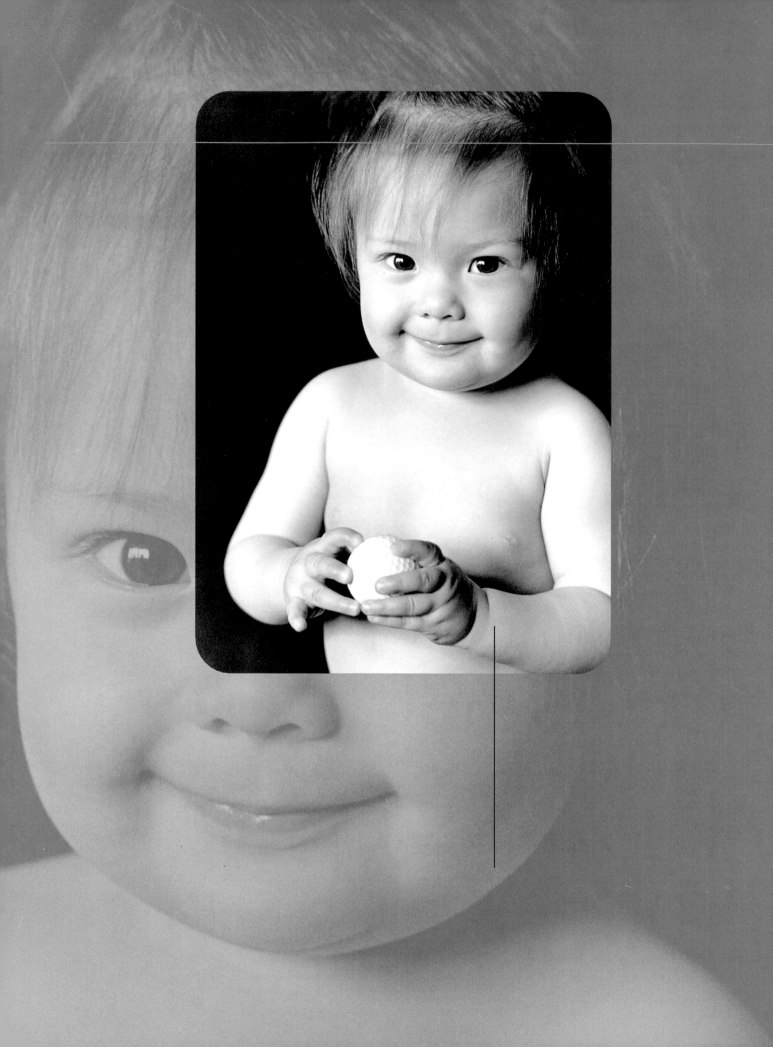

Breakthroughs in Neuroscience—*Why Now?*

Every field of endeavor has peak moments of discovery and opportunity—when past knowledge converges with new needs, new insights, and new technologies to produce stunning advances. For neuroscience, this is one such moment. The last ten years have produced more knowledge about the brain and how it develops than scientists had gleaned in the previous several centuries.

New Research Tools

Why have discoveries in neuroscience advanced so dramatically, capturing the attention of professionals in so many fields? Why now? Certainly, the development of new research tools has been a crucial factor. Dramatic chapters in the history of human exploration have always been prefaced by technological breakthroughs, opening new possibilities, permitting not only material progress but also conceptual leaps and, over time, social change. Some five hundred years ago, new navigational technologies allowed seafarers to find their way to uncharted realms, and at the same time to reframe their contemporaries' thinking about their own world. Today new devices for mapping the human body are allowing new explorations of the brain, and new ways of thinking about how individuals develop and learn.

In the past, investigations of the brain relied heavily on animal studies. Research on humans focused primarily on case studies of people with neurological disorders. Autopsies were also an important source of knowledge; for centuries, most conclusions (and many fallacies) about how people learn and think were premised on observations of the physical size and appearance of different brains and of different parts of the brain. Today, animal studies and autopsies continue to be important sources of knowledge about human anatomy and physiology. But with the help of new technologies, scientists also have numerous ways to study the brains of living people—methods that are designed to be non-invasive. Magnetic Resonance Imaging (MRI) has given neuroscientists a far more detailed view of the brain than was previously possible; a related technology, known as functional MRI, offers new insights into how the brain works. Perhaps the most dramatic advance in brain imaging in recent years has been the Positron Emission

Dramatic chapters in the history of human exploration have always been prefaced by technological breakthroughs.

Tomography or PET scan. The PET scan allows scientists not only to observe brain structure in great detail, but also to record and measure with considerable precision the activity levels of various parts of the brain.

PET scans are powerful tools that can help physicians diagnose and treat a wide range of neurological disorders. But they also provide insight into how normal brains develop in the first years of

The Neuroscientist's Tool Box

Studying Brain Development Before Birth

Today, a number of new techniques are allowing scientists to gain greater understanding of brain development in the prenatal period. For the last two decades, ultrasound imaging has made it possible to get a glimpse of a fetus in the mother's womb. Ultrasound produces computerized images of internal body parts, based on the echoes produced by sound waves. Today, high-resolution ultrasound recordings allow scientists to study and document early brain development—including neural functioning during the prenatal period, and to study fetal behavior. Advances in embryo transplantation have also led to new insights about neural functioning at the earliest stages of life. As a result of these techniques, a view of development is emerging that treats the prenatal period as an adaptive period that is part of a coherent system of development.

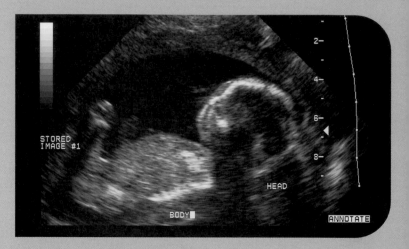

A GLIMPSE OF A FETUS: Ultrasound technology analyzes how sound waves bounce off internal body parts, and then translates this information into a computerized image. This ultrasound shows a fetus in the uterus of a woman who is midway through her pregnancy.

Scanning the Brain

In the past, the only way to get a detailed look at the brain of a living person was to perform surgery. Recent technologies have provided much safer, less invasive ways to create detailed images of the brain, including the Magnetic Resonance Imaging (MRI) scan and the Positron Emission Tomography (PET) scan. Both are used primarily for diagnostic purposes, but have also yielded new insights into how the normal brain develops and functions.

The MRI can produce detailed images of any internal body part. It exposes the body to a magnetic field, and then measures the energy—the nuclear magnetic resonance—that bounces off atoms within the body. Computers then translate these data into detailed images. A related technology, functional MRI, offers insight into how various parts of the body, including specific regions of the brain, work (or do not work). Functional MRI provides information about changes in the volume, flow, or oxygenation of blood that occur as a person undertakes various tasks, including not only motor activities, such as squeezing a hand, but also cognitive tasks, such as speaking or solving a problem.

The PET scan differs from the MRI because it does not just show the brain's structure and function; it also shows how the brain uses energy. To perform a PET scan, scientists inject an individual with a tracer chemical—a compound containing an isotope that gives off particles called positrons. This compound closely resembles glucose, the brain's chief energy source. As a result, the brain is "tricked" into taking up the tracer chemical and trying to use it to fuel its various activities.

This biochemical mimicry has proven immensely useful. By using a special camera that is sensitive to positrons, scientists can visualize not only the fine structures of the brain, but also the level of activity that is taking place in its various parts. That is, they can look at color-coded, cross-sectional images to see how rapidly different parts of the brain take up and try to use the tracer substance. In the process, they can zoom in very precisely on specific parts of the brain; the most up-to-date positron cameras can capture 47 "slices" of the brain at the same time. In this way, neuroscientists can record and quantify a vast amount of information about the structure and activity of a particular brain; they can use these data to create models of brain function. In addition to measuring the brain's activity level, PET scans can also be used to record and measure other aspects of brain function, including blood flow to various parts of the brain, oxygen utilization, protein synthesis, and the release and binding of specialized substances called neurotransmitters.

BRAIN AT WORK: A PET scan shows not only the structure, but also the activity level (metabolic rate), of various parts of the brain. At the time this PET scan was performed, the part of the brain that appears in red was most active.
Source: H.T. Chugani.

Because they require the injection of a tracer compound, PET scans cannot be considered entirely "non-invasive" procedures. But because many children undergo PET scans when neurological problems are suspected or diagnosed, researchers have at their disposal a wide range of data that they can use to draw conclusions about normal development. These data have allowed some insight into the relationship between the developing brain and the environment.

Looking at Brain Waves

The PET scan is the most sophisticated tool now available for studying human brain function, but cannot be used for research purposes with children too young to give informed consent. Other less invasive procedures are more appropriate for research involving young children, and have yielded a great deal of insight into normal brain development. The electroencephalogram (EEG) detects and records brain waves, and can be used to study how the brain reacts to various environmental factors, such as comforting care or stressful conditions. By correlating EEG

Continues on next page

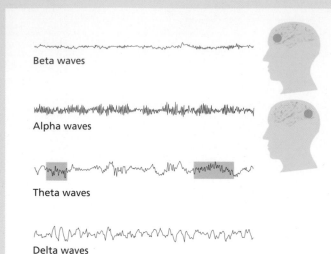

GRAPHING BRAIN WAVES: An electrocephalograph (EEG) detects and graphs brain waves. Four types of brain waves are associated with different parts of the brain and with different states: alert wakefulness (beta); relaxed wakefulness (alpha); the onset of sleep (theta); and deep sleep or coma (delta).

Beta waves

Alpha waves

Theta waves

Delta waves

readings with videotapes of children engaged in various activities, scientists can draw conclusions about the effects of particular events or interactions on the brain's electrical activity. In the past, the EEG also had an "invasive" aspect, since a subject's head had to be slightly scratched to properly attach the electrodes. Recently, neuroscientists developed caps lined with special sponges that allow EEG monitoring of babies and young children without any discomfort.

Analyzing Brain Chemistry

Another significant non-invasive way to study brain development is the analysis of a steroid hormone known as cortisol, which is contained in saliva. Because levels of cortisol in saliva rise when stress increases, a simple saliva test is a fairly accurate way to gauge the impact of adverse conditions on the brain's biochemistry.

Excess cortisol can destroy brain cells and lessen synapse density in some parts of the brain; chronically high levels of cortisol have been associated with some developmental delays and neurological impairments.

Scientists also have new ways to study serotonin, a neurotransmitter that plays a crucial role in brain function. Too much or too little serotonin can affect cognitive and emotional functioning. For example, high levels of serotonin have been associated with autistic spectrum disorders, and low levels with aggression. New techniques have also been developed to study genetic defects that affect the production of serotonin and other biochemical substances needed for normal brain function.

Looking at Children and Families

Less specialized technologies also play a role in generating new knowledge about brain development. Today, many parents in virtually every socioeconomic and ethnic group have access to videotape equipment, at least on special occasions such as children's birthdays. Experts on child development have taken advantage of parents' videotapes to study variations in development. Not only parents, but also researchers frequently use video to study caregiver-child interactions over time.

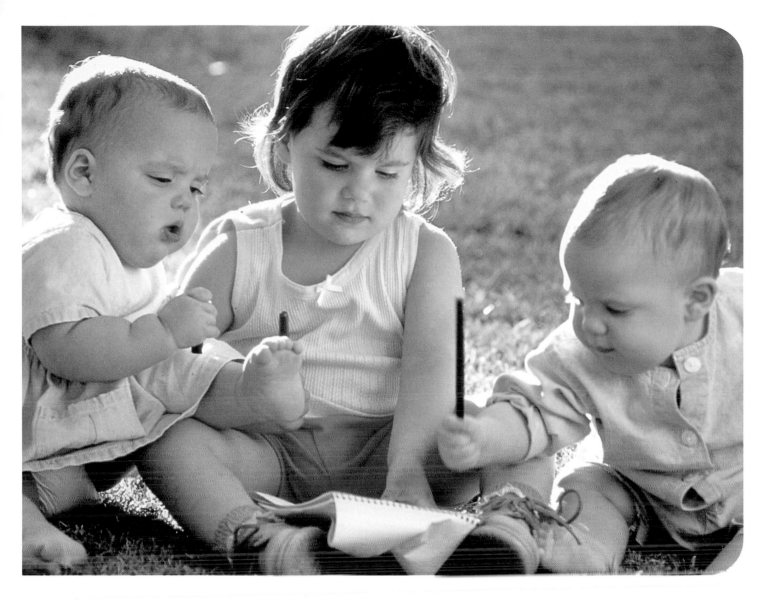

life. For example, by studying the PET scans of infants and toddlers of various ages, scientists can see which parts of the brain are particularly active—that is, undergoing intensive development—at each stage. They can observe closely which parts of the brain are associated with particular activities or are affected by different types of stimulation. And they can draw conclusions about patterns of brain development and neurological functioning that tend to be similar or variable for different individuals.

In short, brain scans and other technologies have made it possible to investigate—and get a glimpse of—the brain's intricate circuitry and how it evolves. Neuroscientists have also greatly expanded our understanding of brain chemistry, and in

particular the effects of various environmental factors on the brain. At the same time, they have gained insight into the nature of brain dysfunction.

The Context for Recent Brain Research

Technological breakthroughs never occur in a vacuum. Without a favorable social and ideological context, and without a widely shared perception of need, the sustained research and development needed to perfect new technologies rarely take place. Or, even if they do, the new knowledge or new possibilities that they generate may not

The Quiet Crisis

In the 1994 report entitled *Starting Points*, the Carnegie Task Force on Meeting the Needs of Our Youngest Children described the quiet crisis that faces infants and toddlers and their families. *Starting Points* reported that "of the 12 million children under the age of three in the United States today, a staggering number are affected by one or more risk factors that make a healthy development more difficult." In the three years since *Starting Points* appeared, there have been improvements in some areas. For example, teen pregnancy rates are gradually declining, and immunization rates are rising. But many risk factors remain:

- Seven percent of babies are born with low birthweight (less than 5.5 pounds), and are therefore at greater risk for disabilities and death. For children born to smokers, the rate is nearly 12 percent.
- One-fifth of all expectant mothers, and one-third of African American, Latina, and American Indian expectant mothers, receive no prenatal care in the first trimester of pregnancy. Four percent of all expectant mothers receive no care at all or receive care very late in their pregnancies.
- One-fourth of all two year olds in the U.S.—more than one million children—do not receive their full series of recommended immunizations.
- A total of 2.2 million children under the age of three have no health insurance either through employer coverage or Medicaid.
- The incidence of child abuse and neglect has increased dramatically over the last decade. The number rose from 1.4 million in 1986 to more than 2.8 million in 1993. (This is an estimate of actual cases of abuse and neglect, not just reported cases.) During the same period, the number of children who were seriously injured quadrupled.
- Each year, some 21,000 newborns are abandoned or become boarder babies, remaining in hospitals after they are medically ready to leave.
- The U.S. has the highest teen pregnancy rate among developed countries. About 1 million teenagers become pregnant each year; 80 percent of those pregnancies are unintended and almost 50 percent end in abortions.

become widely known or exploited. Brain research has been stimulated, in part, by the search for better ways to help individuals with neurological disorders. But today, intensive interest in early brain development also reflects growing concern about the status of children in America—not only their academic achievement, but also their health, safety, and overall well-being.

Two decades of productive research in the fields of child development, education, and cognitive science, and the evaluation of early intervention and school reform initiatives, have generated substantial knowledge about the kinds of initiatives and programs that are likely to work. Research has consistently shown that high quality child care and early education can boost children's chances for later success in school. But today, most American preschoolers who are in out-of-home care—particularly infants and toddlers—are in settings of poor to mediocre quality.[1] Educators estimate that millions of American children—at least a third—enter kindergarten unprepared to benefit from the kinds of instruction and interactions they encounter in their classrooms.[2] Poor school performance is foreshadowed by below-average performance on measures of cognitive and social functioning during the preschool years.[3]

These facts are particularly alarming in view of considerable evidence that by the time they are eight years old, children are launched into trajectories that largely determine their academic futures. Researchers have been able to predict the likelihood of students' dropping out of high school based on their academic performance and social adjustment in the third grade.[4] Some researchers have predicted drop-out patterns before children even enter school, based on the quality of care and support they receive in the first years of life. L. Alan Sroufe and his colleagues at the University of Minnesota, who have followed hundreds of children over two decades, report that children's achievement at age 16 can be predicted based on the level of support they receive in their preschool years.[5] Finally, a growing body of research shows that when children do not get a good start in the early years, later remediation becomes much more difficult and costly.[6]

Given these findings, there is growing frustration with educational investments and educational research that focus primarily on school-age children, and learning strategies that begin only when children reach the age of five. There is greater recognition that if, as a society, we fail to meet the needs of our youngest children, none of our strategies for teaching them later will be as effective. Many Americans from all walks of life are coming to the conclusion that to improve achievement and help our students solve the complex problems they will encounter on a daily basis in the next century, we as a nation must support efforts that expand and apply the most fundamental knowledge available to us about how children develop (or fail to develop) the capacity to learn and to thrive in a variety of settings. More and more decision makers in diverse fields are coming to believe that efforts to recast policy and reconsider the best use of public resources must begin with clearheaded thinking about young children's brains.

New Interest in the Brain Across Diverse Disciplines

The conviction that the early years are crucial is provoking, across a wide range of disciplines, greater interest in neuroscience in general and early brain development in particular. Professionals in education and the human services are becoming more receptive to new knowledge about human brain development. Developmental psychologists and anthropologists are turning to neuroscience for insight into the relationship between the workings of the human mind and the evolution of different cultures; moreover, social scientists and neurobiologists are finding many commonalities in their findings. Leaders in the broadcast and print media are recognizing the far-reaching implications of recent brain research, and are taking steps to make it available to the public. There are new opportunities for collaboration, and a greater commitment by neuroscientists to making their work accessible and meaningful to nonspecialists.

In short, working across disciplines, researchers, practitioners, and policy makers in diverse fields are engaged in an active, exciting effort to rethink the brain, and to apply new knowledge and ideas that can support the healthy development and well-being of children. As researchers amass a growing body of vital information about the brain, the public is beginning to get the message.

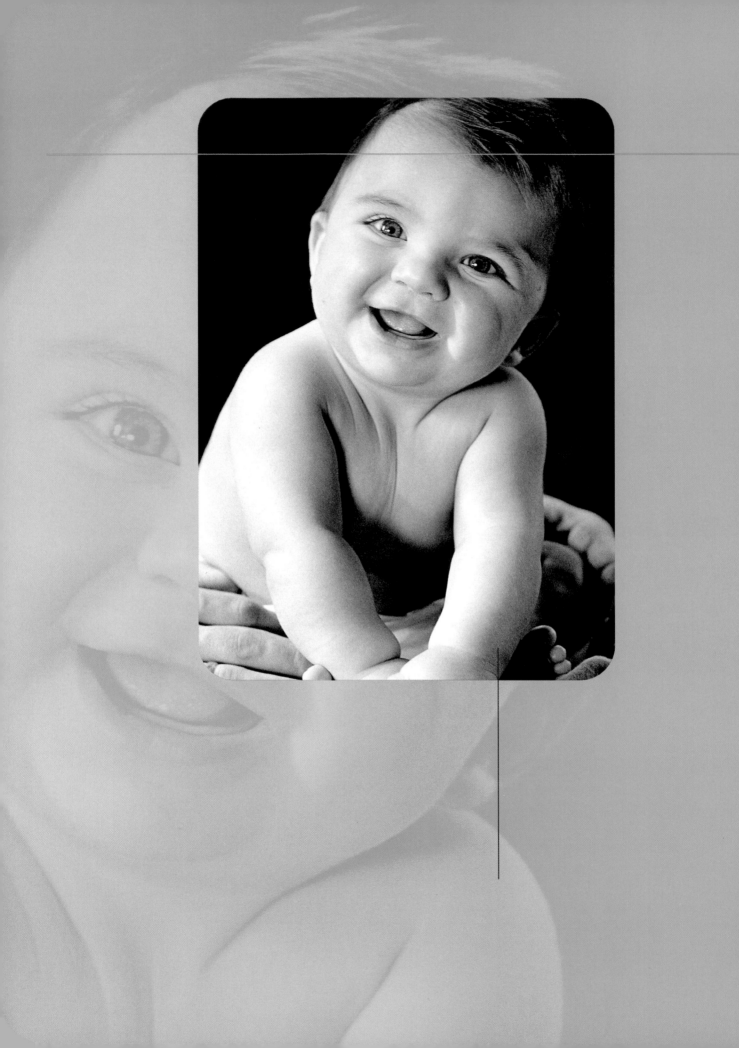

What Have We *Learned?*

The research presented at the June 1996 conference pointed to five key lessons that have the potential to reframe research, policy, and practice in diverse fields committed to improving results for children and families.

1. | **Human development hinges on the interplay between nature and nurture.** Much of our thinking about the brain has been dominated by old assumptions—that the genes we are born with determine how our brains develop, and that, in turn, how our brains develop determines how we interact with the world. These assumptions are not often stated in such explicit terms, but they underlie many conventional notions about why people and cultures are so different from each other. In some cases, they have been used to justify fatalistic and fallacious assertions that certain groups or individuals are bound to fail.[7]

Recent brain research challenges these assumptions. Neuroscientists have shown that throughout the entire process of development—beginning even before birth—the brain is affected by environmental conditions, including the kind of nourishment, care, surroundings, and stimulation an individual receives. The impact of the environment is dramatic and specific, not merely influencing the general direction of development, but actually affecting how the intricate circuitry of the human brain is "wired." And because every individual is exposed to different experiences, no two brains are wired the same way. Of the nearly six billion people alive on the earth today, no two individuals have the same brain. Even identical twins, born with the same genetic endowment, will develop differently based on how and when various environmental factors affect the development of their brains.

The Impact of the Environment

To be sure, genes play an important role, endowing every individual with a particular set of predispositions. (Indeed, roughly 60 percent of genes in the human body are dedicated to brain development.) In recent years, geneticists have made significant breakthroughs in their understanding of the relationship between genes and human behavior. For example, they are beginning to identify specific genes that appear to predispose an individual toward certain traits such as a bashful or outgoing social style. But they acknowledge that genetic endowment is only part of the equation; it is the dynamic relationship between nature and nurture that shapes human development.

Parents often notice that children have different temperaments. From birth, some appear to be more outgoing and adaptable; others tend to be more withdrawn and slow to warm up.[8] To be sure, genes play a role in determining temperament; but as researchers have shown, even before birth, the intrauterine environment can have a decisive influence on development, including temperamental differences in children. As infants grow, their predispositions are vitally influenced by a wide range of environmental factors, including not only the physical but also the social and emotional settings.

Neuroscientists stress the fact that interaction with the environment is not simply an interesting feature of brain development; it is an absolute

The Brain in Brief

Brain Structure

The brain is part of the central nervous system, and plays a decisive role in controlling many bodily functions, including both voluntary activities (such as walking or speaking) and involuntary ones (such as breathing or blinking).

The brain has two hemispheres, and each hemisphere has four lobes. Each of these lobes has numerous folds. These folds do not all mature at the same time. The chemicals that foster brain development are released in waves; as a result, different areas of the brain evolve in a predictable sequence. The timing of these developmental changes explains, in part, why there are "prime times" for certain kinds of learning and development.

Different parts of the brain control different kinds of functions. Most of the activities that we think of as "brain work," like thinking, planning, or remembering, are handled by the cerebral cortex, the uppermost, ridged portion of the brain. Other parts of the brain also play a role in memory and learning, including the thalamus, hippocampus, amygdala, and basal forebrain. The hypothalamus and amygdala, as well as other parts of the brain, are also important in reacting to stress and controlling emotions.

Brain Cells

Of course, the basic building blocks of the brain are much smaller than an illustration could show. They are the specialized nerve cells that make up the central nervous system—neurons. The nerve cells proliferate before birth. In fact, a fetus' brain produces roughly twice as many neurons as it will eventually need—a safety margin that gives newborns the best possible chance of coming into the world with healthy brains. Most of the excess neurons are shed in utero. At birth, an infant has roughly 100 billion brain cells.

Every neuron has an axon (usually only one)—an "output" fiber that sends impulses to other neurons; each neuron also has many dendrites—short hairlike "input" fibers that receive impulses from other neurons. In this way, neurons are perfectly constructed to form connections.

As a child grows, the number of neurons remains relatively stable, but each cell grows, becoming bigger and heavier. The proliferation of dendrites accounts for some of this growth. The dendrites branch out, forming "dendrite trees" that can receive signals from many other neurons.

Connections among Brain Cells

At birth, the human brain is in a remarkably unfinished state. Most of its 100 billion neurons are not yet connected in networks. Forming and reinforcing these connections are the key tasks of early brain development.

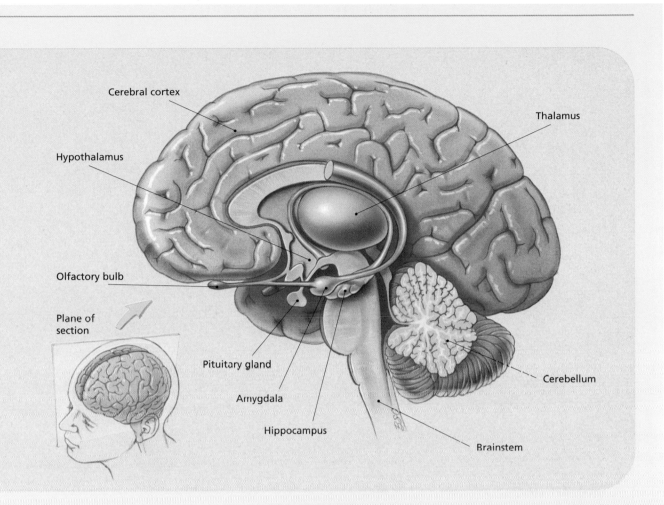

Cerebral cortex

Thalamus

Hypothalamus

Olfactory bulb

Plane of section

Pituitary gland

Amygdala

Hippocampus

Cerebellum

Brainstem

AN ADULT BRAIN: This side view shows one hemisphere. Different parts of the brain control different kinds of functions. Most of the activities we think of as "brain work," like thinking, planning, or remembering, are handled by the cerebral cortex.

Connections among neurons are formed as the growing child experiences the surrounding world and forms attachments to parents, family members, and other caregivers.

In the first decade of life, a child's brain forms trillions of connections or synapses. Axons hook up with dendrites, and chemicals called neurotransmitters facilitate the passage of impulses across the resulting synapses. Each individual neuron may be connected to as many as 15,000 other neurons, forming a network of neural pathways that is immensely complex. This elaborate network is sometimes referred to as the brain's "wiring" or "circuitry."

In the early years, children's brains form twice as many synapses as they will eventually need. If these synapses are used repeatedly in a child's day-to-day life, they are reinforced and become part of the brain's permanent circuitry. If they are not used repeatedly, or often enough, they are eliminated. In this way, experience plays a crucial role in "wiring" a young child's brain.

Rethinking the Brain

How a brain develops depends on the genes you are born with.

How a brain develops hinges on a complex interplay between the genes you're born with and the experiences you have.

The experiences you have before age three have a limited impact on later development.

Early experiences have a decisive impact on the architecture of the brain, and on the nature and extent of adult capacities.

A secure relationship with a primary caregiver creates a favorable context for early development and learning.

Early interactions don't just create a context; they directly affect the way the brain is "wired."

Brain development is linear: the brain's capacity to learn and change grows steadily as an infant progresses toward adulthood.

Brain development is non-linear: there are prime times for acquiring different kinds of knowledge and skills.

A toddler's brain is much less active than the brain of a college student.

By the time children reach age three, their brains are twice as active as those of adults. Activity levels drop during adolescence.

requirement. It is built into the process of development, beginning within days of conception. From an evolutionary standpoint, there is a very good reason for this. The demands on the human brain are immense—one is tempted to say, unthinkable. In addition to controlling and monitoring all of the body's vital functions, this single organ must receive and process information about the world from the millions of sensory receptors reporting from the body surface and the internal organs; it must factor in past experience; it must then respond and adapt appropriately. In short, it must learn continuously and intensively. Carrying out these tasks requires billions of brain cells (or neurons), and trillions of connections (or synapses) among them. Because this challenge is so overwhelming, the brain has a unique way of developing that sets it apart from every other organ in the human body. Gradually creating and organizing billions of brain cells in a predetermined manner during early childhood would demand more information (in the form of genetic coding) than the body could possibly dedicate to this purpose. Nature solved this problem by evolving a more economical system. The developing brain produces many times more neurons and more synapses than it will eventually need. Most of the extra neurons are shed by the time a baby is born. The brain continues to grow in size, however, as each neuron expands; by adulthood, the brain will quadruple in weight. While the number of neurons remains stable, the number of synapses increases markedly in the first three years.

How are these connections formed? Neurons are designed for efficient connectivity. Every neuron has an axon, which sends electrical signals to other neurons, and numerous hairlike structures called dendrites which receive incoming signals. A synapse is produced when the axon of one neuron connects with the dendrite of another. Transmission of an electrical signal across this hookup requires a neurotransmitter chemical such as serotonin, dopamine, or the endorphins. The resulting connections are profuse: in the early years of life, each neuron forms up to 15,000 synapses.

The brain development of infants and toddlers proceeds at a staggering pace. By the age of two, the number of synapses reaches adult levels; by age three, a child's brain has 1,000 trillion synapses—about twice as many as her pediatrician's. This number holds steady throughout the first decade of life. In this way a young child's brain becomes super-dense.

These conclusions are not based on mere speculation. As early as the 1970s—ancient history

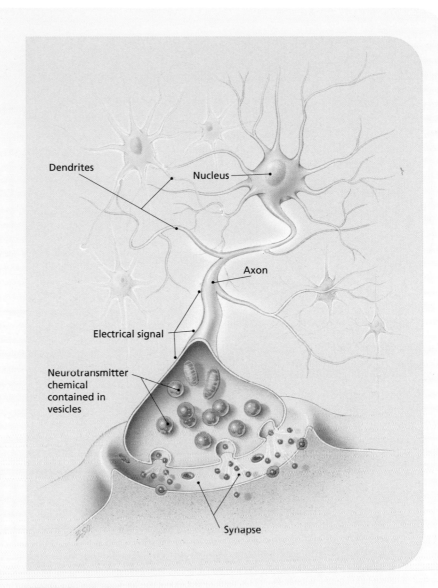

READY TO LEARN: Making connections is a neuron's mission. The axon of one neuron hooks up with the dendrite of another to form a synapse. Neurotransmitters enable electrical impulses to travel across the synapse.

from the neuroscientist's perspective—Peter Huttenlocher at the University of Chicago began counting synapses in the frontal cortex. He observed that children's brains have many more synapses than adults' brains, and that the density of synapses remains high throughout the first decade of life.[9] After this, there is a gradual decline in synapse density; by the time a child reaches late adolescence, half of all the synapses in the brain have been discarded, leaving about 500 trillion—a

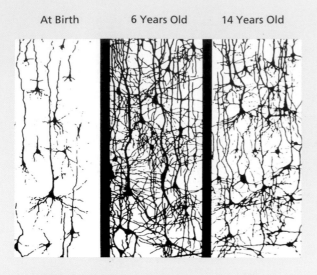

At Birth 6 Years Old 14 Years Old

SYNAPTIC DENSITY: Synapses are created with astonishing speed in the first three years of life. For the rest of the first decade, children's brains have twice as many synapses as adults' brains.
Drawings supplied by H.T. Chugani.

number that remains relatively constant for the rest of the life cycle.

Brain development is, then, a process of pruning: the brain selectively eliminates excess synapses. In fact, the brain appears to be actively producing and eliminating synapses throughout life. In the first three years, production far outpaces elimination; for the rest of the first decade, production and elimination are roughly balanced; and beginning in early adolescence, elimination is clearly the dominant process. In this way, as a child grows, an overabundance of connections gives way to a complex, powerful system of neural pathways.

But how does the brain "know" which connections to keep and which to discard? This is where early experience plays a crucial role. When some kind of stimulus activates a neural pathway, all the synapses that form that pathway receive and store a chemical signal. Repeated activation increases the strength of that signal. When the signal reaches a threshold level (which differs for different areas of the brain), something extraordinary happens to that synapse. It becomes exempt from elimina-

tion—and retains its protected status into adulthood. Scientists do not yet fully understand the mechanism by which this occurs; they conjecture that the electrical activity produced when neural pathways are activated gives rise to chemical changes that stabilize the synapse.

These findings confirm that brain development is a "use it or lose it" process. As pruning accelerates in the second decade of life, those synapses that have been reinforced by virtue of repeated experience tend to become permanent; the synapses that were not used often enough in the early years tend to be eliminated. In this way the experiences—positive or negative—that young children have in the first years of life influence how their brains will be wired as adults.

The dynamic process of producing and eliminating synapses offers clear benefits. For example, it enables young children to adapt readily to many different kinds of conditions and settings. It helps children who grow up in a setting where survival hinges on efficient hunting to acquire the necessary perceptual and physical skills, while enabling children who grow up in an urban environment to develop the capacity to filter out certain kinds of stimulation.

To be sure, maintaining large numbers of synapses requires considerable energy. Using PET scan technology, Harry Chugani and his colleagues at Michigan Children's Hospital, Wayne State University, have documented the fact that in the early years, the human brain has a significantly higher metabolic rate (as measured by its utilization of glucose) than it will have later in life, presumably due to the profusion of connections being formed in the brains of young children.

Indeed, based on measurements of glucose utilization, Chugani has found that the brain development that takes place before a baby's first birthday is more rapid and extensive than neurobiologists

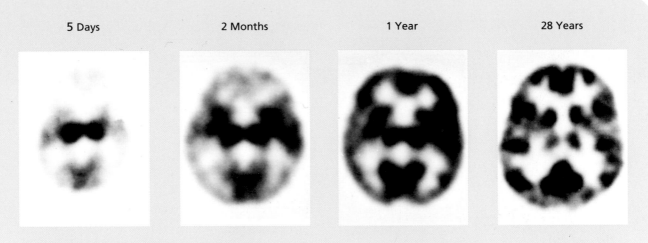

| 5 Days | 2 Months | 1 Year | 28 Years |

RAPID EARLY DEVELOPMENT: These PET scans suggest that the brain of a one year old more closely resembles an adult's brain than a newborn's.

Source: H.T. Chugani

previously suspected. A newborn's brain is in a largely subcortical state; its cerebral cortex—the part of the brain responsible for complex cognitive functions like language and spatial orientation—is relatively dormant. By the time the candle is lit on the baby's first birthday cake, the brain has achieved a highly cortical state. But the cortex is not the only region of the brain to mature quickly. PET scans show that by the age of one, a baby's brain qualitatively resembles that of a normal young adult. This transformation corresponds to the dramatic changes that parents and other people who care for babies witness in the first year, as newborns progress with incredible speed from virtually helpless beings to children who are starting to reason, to walk and talk, to form intentions and carry them out, and to enjoy interactions with a variety of people, pets, and objects.

By the age of two, toddlers' brains are as active as those of adults. The metabolic rate keeps rising, and by the age of three, the brains of children are two and a half times more active than the brains of adults—and they stay that way throughout the first decade of life. Compared with adult brains, children's brains also have higher levels of some neuro-transmitters, which play an important role in the formation of synapses. All of these factors—synapse density, glucose utilization, and the level of some neurotransmitters—remain high throughout the first decade of life, and begin to decline only with puberty. This suggests that young children—particularly infants and toddlers—are biologically primed for learning.[10]

The pruning process proceeds at a rapid pace in the second decade of life, but does not occur at the same rate in all parts of the brain. Fewer changes

By the age of three, the brains of children are two and a half times more active than the brains of adults—and they stay that way throughout the first decade of life.

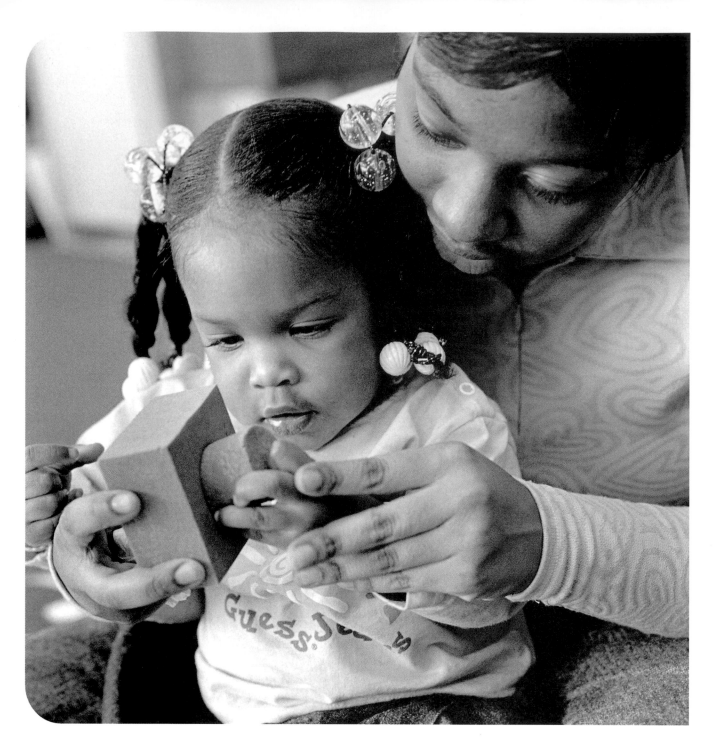

are seen in the more "hard-wired" areas of the brain, such as the brainstem, that control such involuntary functions as respiration. In contrast, the most dramatic pruning has been observed in the cerebral cortex. As this part of the brain develops, roughly 33 synapses are eliminated every second—suggesting that the developing brain responds constantly and swiftly to ongoing conditions that promote (or inhibit) learning.[11]

Connectivity is a crucial feature of brain development, because the neural pathways formed during the early years carry signals and allow us to process information throughout our lives. How, and how well, we think and learn—both as children and as adults—has a great deal to do with the extent and nature of these connections. Researchers have measured the level of brain activity required for different tasks, and have found that when individuals address more difficult problems, brain activity surges. But if a problem is solved easily, changes in brain activity are virtually undetectable.[12] This reflects the role of connectivity: when experience and learning have created efficient neural pathways, signals travel easily among them and the processing of information requires relatively little effort.

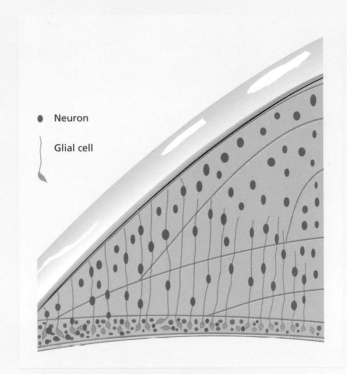

CORTICAL CELL MIGRATION: Cortical neurons (above) develop in the deepest layer of the immature cortex and travel up glial cells ("cortical ladders"). The information they pick up from other neurons they pass along the way determines their identity.

A CORTICAL LADDER: A double exposed photograph (right) of neuronal migration up a glial cell.
Source: *Journal of Neuroscience* (reprinted with permission).

The Development of the Cortex

Pasko Rakic and his colleagues at Yale University have found that the cerebral cortex is vulnerable to environmental influence from its earliest stages of development—within days of conception. By studying macaque monkeys, whose brain development closely parallels that of humans, Rakic and his colleagues have found that as a fetus develops, brain cells have to find their way up the cerebral wall, sliding up elongated cells called glial fibers until they reach their precise position within the cerebral cortex. The sequence and timing of this process must adhere to a very precise schedule if normal development is to occur. As a cell climbs this cortical "ladder," it comes into contact with the numerous cells that it passes on its rise to the top. This contact activates various genes that define the cell's identity, location, and mission. But if anything interrupts or sidetracks this journey—such as exposure to adverse environmental conditions or a lack of nutrition—the effects can be devastating.[13]

Often cells that go astray will die before any harm is done. But, as Rakic observes, if cells end up in the wrong place at the wrong time and form inappropriate synapses, the result may be a neurological disorder such as severe infantile epilepsy, autism, or schizophrenia. The delicate nature of this cell migration process explains, in part, why

"The Ecological Brain"—An Anthropologist's View

From Bradd Shore, *Culture in Mind: Cognition, Culture, and the Problem of Meaning.* New York: Oxford University Press, 1996. (Reprinted with the permission of Oxford University Press.)

The implications are, quite literally, mind-bending. At birth, the human brain weights a mere 25 percent of its eventual adult weight. This is a curious state of affairs for the brainiest of the primates. A macaque, by contrast, is born with a brain that is 60 percent of its adult weight. Its neural growth has already slowed dramatically while still in utero. Even our closest primate relation, the chimpanzee, is born with about 45 percent of its brain weight already developed, and its brain growth slows down shortly after birth. Chimps mature both physically and socially years ahead of their human cousins.

Among primates, only the human brain continues to grow at fetal rates after birth, and the frantic pace of this postpartum neural building boom continues for the first two years of life before it begins to show any signs of abating. The cortex's natural insulation, the fatty myelin sheath that grows about the axons and permits efficient connection of electrical impulses, is not completely formed until about the sixth year of life. Only at puberty is the physical maturation of the human brain complete. After that, neural development continues throughout life. But this is, strictly speaking, more a matter of "mind" than of brain.

This delayed maturation of the human nervous system is paralleled by a general developmental retardation of the human child compared with other primates. Humans also show a tendency to both physiological and behavioral neoteny, retaining juvenile traits in adult forms of both anatomy (i.e., head-body ratio) and behavior (i.e., playfulness).

This combination of premature birth and retarded development means that fully three-quarters of the human brain develops outside the womb, in direct relationship with an external environment. Evolution has equipped our species with an "ecological brain," dependent throughout its life on environmental input. This is a factor of extraordinary significance for cultural anthropology and cognitive psychology alike.

substance abuse, poor nutrition, or exposure to radiation can have a long-lasting or permanent impact on a developing fetus.[14]

By elaborating processes such as cell migration, neuroscience has given us a much more specific picture of the risks that threaten early brain development, and we know precisely when those risks are highest. For example, a fetus that is exposed to cocaine or to radiation on the fourteenth day after conception is likely to have a different (and worse) outcome than a fetus exposed on the thirtieth day. These findings have far-reaching implications for prenatal preventive care. Indeed, they suggest the need for early parent education, since many expectant mothers do not know that they are carrying a child until well after the days of highest risk have passed.

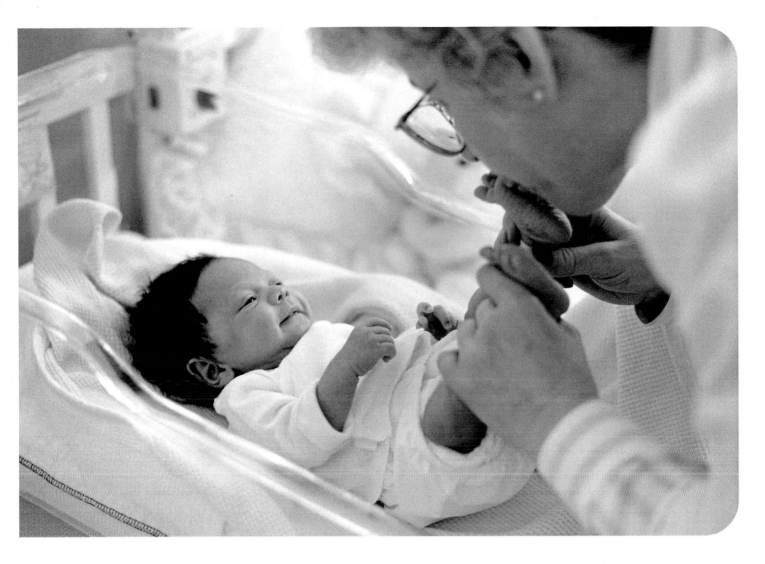

Humans and Other Primates

Some of the research cited thus far comes from animal studies, and to be sure the neurobiology of animals—even other primates—differs significantly from that of human beings. But compared to the brains of other species, the human brain is even more primed to respond to experience and the environment. Bradd Shore of Emory University emphasizes, in a recent book on cognition and culture, that compared with other species, humans are born with remarkably undeveloped brains—"a curious state of affairs for the brainiest of the primates."[15] Other primates, including the macaque monkeys studied by many neuroscientists, come into the world with brains that are much further along in their own development trajectories: at birth, their brains are closer to their eventual adult weight and show less dramatic growth. Among primates, only the human brain enters the world in such an unfinished state. Indeed, in humans the great preponderance of brain development takes place outside the womb, in direct relationship with the external environment. In short, to a greater extent than other species, humans have brains that are dependent on environmental input.

But experience does not begin at birth. A growing body of evidence (from studies of humans) confirms that even before birth, brain development and perceptual learning are affected by experience, including a fetus' own sensory and motor experiences. Ultrasound recordings show that the neurons that develop in utero begin driving an infant's limbs

Day-to-Day Care of Young Children's Brains

Recent research on early brain development and school readiness suggest the following broad guidelines for the care of young children:

- Ensure health, safety, and good nutrition — Seek regular prenatal care; breast feed if possible; make sure your child has regular check-ups and timely immunizations; safety-proof the places where children play; and use a car seat whenever your child is travelling in a car.

- Develop a warm, caring relationship with children — Show them that you care deeply about them. Express joy in who they are. Help them feel safe and secure.

- Respond to children's cues and clues — Notice their rhythms and moods, even in the first days and weeks of life. Respond to children when they are upset as well as when they are happy. Try to understand what children are feeling, what they are telling you (in words or actions), and what they are trying to do. Hold and touch them; play with them in a way that lets you follow their lead. Move in when children want to play, and pull back when they seem to have had enough stimulation.

- Recognize that each child is unique — Keep in mind that from birth, children have different temperaments, that they grow at their own pace, and that this pace varies from child to child. At the same time, have positive expectations about what children can do and hold onto the belief that every child can succeed.

- Talk, read, and sing to children — Surround them with language. Maintain an ongoing conversation with them about what you and they are doing. Sing to them, play music, tell stories and read books. Ask toddlers and preschoolers to guess what will come next in a story. Play word games. Ask toddlers and preschoolers questions that require more than a yes or no answer, like "What do you think...?" Ask children to picture things that have happened in the past or might happen in the future. Provide reading and writing materials, including crayons and paper, books, magazines, and toys. These are key pre-reading experiences.

as early as at seven weeks of gestation. In his remarks at the conference, Myron A. Hofer of Columbia University and the New York State Psychiatric Institute, wondered aloud why there should be so much fetal activity so early in pregnancy, in view of the fact that this activity is not needed to help the fetus adapt to the perfectly suitable intrauterine environment. He concludes that a key function of early fetal activity is to aid the process of constructing the brain, so that from the very start, experience can act on the brain's develop-ment. Experimental data confirm that learning can take place in utero. Studies have shown, for example, that newborns will show a preference (by sucking on a pacifier more intensely) for sounds that mimic the mother's voice as it was heard in utero.[16]

All of this evidence—and a great deal more that is beyond the scope of this report—leads to a single conclusion: how humans develop and learn depends critically and continually on the interplay between nature (an individual's genetic endowment) and nurture (the nutrition, surroundings, care, stimulation, and teaching that are provided or withheld). The roles of nature and nurture in determining intelligence and emotional resilience should not be weighted quantitatively; genetic and environmental factors have a more dynamic, quali-

- **Encourage safe exploration and play** — Give children opportunities to move around, explore and play (and be prepared to step in if they are at risk of hurting themselves or others). Allow them to explore relationships as well. Arrange for children to spend time with children of their own age and of other ages. Help them learn to solve the conflicts that inevitably arise.

- **Use discipline to teach** — Talk to children about what they seem to be feeling and teach them words to describe those feelings. Make it clear that while you might not like they way they are behaving, you love them. Explain the rules and consequences of behavior so children can learn the "whys" behind what you are asking them to do. Tell them what you want them to do, not just what you don't want them to do. Point out how their behavior affects others.

- **Establish routines** — Create routines and rituals for special times during the day like meal time, nap time, and bed time. Try to be predictable so the children know that they can count on you.

- **Become involved in child care and preschool** — Keep in close touch with your children's child care providers or teachers about what they are doing. From time to time, especially during transitions, spend time with your children while they are being cared for by others.

- **Limit television** — Limit the time children spend watching TV shows and videos as well as the type of shows they watch. Make sure that they are watching programs that will teach them things you want them to learn.

- **Take care of yourself** — You can best care for young children when you are cared for as well.

tative interplay that cannot be reduced to a simple equation. Both factors are crucial. New knowledge about brain development should end the "nature or nurture" debate once and for all.

2. | **Early care and nurture have a decisive, long-lasting impact on how people develop, their ability to learn, and their capacity to regulate their own emotions.** Parents and other caregivers have long known that babies thrive when they receive warm, responsive early care; now we are beginning to understand the biological mechanisms that underlie this common knowledge. Responsive caregiving not only meets babies' basic, day-to-day needs for nourishment and warmth, but also takes into account their rhythms, preferences, and moods. The ways that parents, families, and other caregivers relate and respond to young children, and the ways that they mediate their children's contact with the environment, directly affect the formation of neural pathways. We know, for example, that parents tend to mimic and reinforce their infants' positive emotional responses. Interactions like these appear to influence developing patterns of neuronal connectivity.[17]

The Protective Function of Warm, Responsive Care

Recent brain research suggests that warm, responsive care is not only comforting for an infant; it is critical to healthy development. In fact, a strong, secure attachment to a nurturing caregiver appears to have a protective biological function, "immunizing" an infant to some degree against the adverse

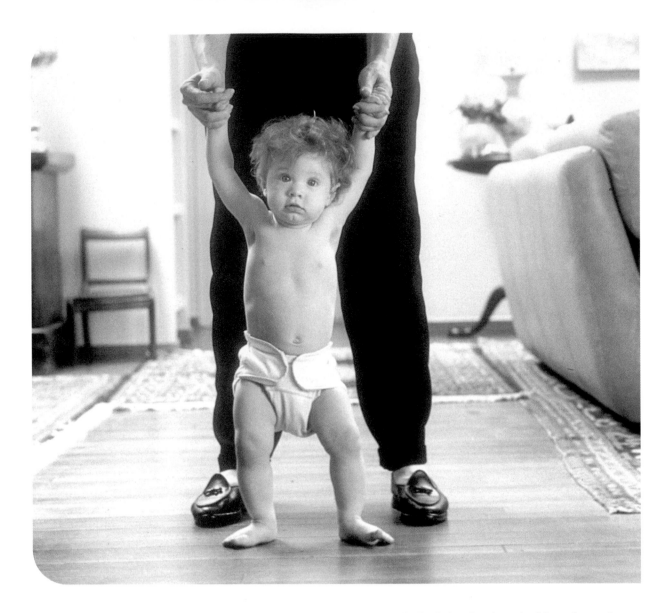

effects of later stress or trauma. These are the implications of research by Megan R. Gunnar of the University of Minnesota, who has gauged children's reactions to stress by measuring the levels of a steroid hormone called cortisol in their saliva. Researchers have known for some time that adverse or traumatic events, whether physical or psychological, can elevate an individual's cortisol level. In turn, cortisol affects metabolism, the immune system, and the brain. Cortisol alters the brain by making it vulnerable to processes that destroy neurons and, just as importantly, by reducing the number of synapses in certain parts of the brain. In this way, stressful or traumatic experiences can indeed undermine neurological development and impair brain function. And in fact, children who have

chronically high levels of cortisol have been shown to experience more developmental delays—cognitive, motor, and social—than other children.[18]

But some children seem to weather stress better than others, and Gunnar's research asks why. Her findings suggest that babies who receive sensitive and nurturing care in their first year of life are less likely than other children to respond to minor stresses by producing cortisol than other children. And when they do respond by producing cortisol, they can more rapidly and efficiently turn off this response. This protective effect has been shown to carry forward to later childhood: elementary school children with histories of secure attachment are less likely to show behavior problems in the face of stress.[19] Specialists in child development have long observed that babies who receive warm, responsive care tend to thrive and to show more resilience later in life. Now neuroscientists are gathering important biological clues about why.

Gunnar's research confirms that early neurological development is shaped not only by physical conditions, but also by an individual's social environment. Indeed, there is mounting evidence that the kind of care infants receive, and the kind of attachments they form with their primary caregivers, have a decisive effect on their regulatory capacities—in particular their emerging ability to display and modulate emotions. In other words, a child's capacity to control emotions appears to hinge, to a significant extent, on biological systems shaped by her early experiences. When a child is abandoned or emotionally neglected very early in life, such brain-mediated functions as empathy, attachment, and affect regulation are often impaired.[20]

The Importance of Attachment

Since neuroscientists now confirm that children are primed for learning in the first few years, parents and other caregivers may feel compelled to expose their babies to a steady flow of information and intellectual stimulation. Should expectant parents recite the multiplication table to their unborn babies? Should child care providers encourage toddlers to memorize many facts and figures? The answer is: measures like these are unnecessary. Children learn in the context of important relationships. The best way to help very young children grow into curious, confident, able learners is to give them warm, consistent care so that they can form secure attachments to those who care for them. Paying attention to an infant's moods, knowing when he needs comfort rather than stimulation (or vice versa), mimicking a baby's trills and "beebee-

Early neurological development is shaped not only by physical conditions, but also by an individual's social environment.

bees," or following a toddler's lead as she invents a new version of peekaboo—these interactions are all part of responsive care, and do far more to boost later learning than, say, flash cards or tapes of the ABCs.

The psychological and psychoanalytic literatures contain a substantial body of work, notably classic studies by John Bowlby, emphasizing the importance and complexity of an infant's attachment to her mother or primary caregiver, and the traumatic effects of the experience of loss or long-term separation from the mother. But children are not only affected by a breach of attachment; research launched in the 1970s that followed children over time showed that qualitative differences in attachment can have long-term psychological consequences. Alan Sroufe and his colleagues provide strong evidence of the link between early care and a child's later capacity to connect well with others. For example, young children who receive highly erratic care are more prone to becoming very dependent and anxious later in life; children who receive persistently unresponsive care are more likely than other children to shut down emotionally and to act in ways that keep others at a distance.[21] In contrast, children who receive consistent, responsive care in the first years of life are more likely to develop strong social skills.

Following Children Through the Decades

Neurobiologists tell us that the experiences children have in the first years of life affect their abilities and behaviors throughout childhood and into adulthood. The evidence they produce is impressive. But do real children in real families develop in the ways that brain scientists predict? Do insecure attachments or adverse environmental conditions actually show up, years later, as learning disabilities, emotional distress, or behavior problems? To know for sure, one would have to study a large number of children, beginning before birth and continuing over at least two decades.

That is precisely what Byron Egeland, L. Alan Sroufe and their colleagues at the University of Minnesota have done. Since 1975, they have conducted a long-term study of high-risk families. Known as the Minnesota Parent-Child Project, the research project began with 267 women in the last trimester of their first pregnancies whose incomes placed them below the poverty line; two decades later, 180 children were still participating in the study. Over the years, the research team carried out frequent and varied assessments of both mothers and children, separately and together, and documented the contexts in which they lived. The assessments have included objective psychological tests, interviews, questionnaires, and observations of child behavior and mother-child interactions.

More recently, researchers such as Alicia Lieberman of the University of California at San Francisco and Charles Zeanah of the Louisiana State University School of Medicine, have stressed the long-term impact of infant attachment, underscoring the importance of "goodness of fit" between parents and their infant, and describing techniques that can help them become well attuned to each other. They also note that infants are capable of becoming attached to more than one caregiver, but do develop, from a very young age, an internal hierarchy or "order of preference."[22] Researchers such as Kyle Pruett of Yale University are also beginning to consider fathers' contributions to children's well-being, and the influence on early development of fathers' ways of making eye contact, playing with children, and using vocalization. There has been some research on fathers who are their young children's primary caregivers, but more work is needed in this area.

Recent brain research deepens our understanding of the effects of different patterns of attachment and, moving beyond the psychological, documents the biological factors that help to explain these effects. Myron Hofer's research over three decades bridges the findings of psychologists and biologists, illuminating a range of biological processes underlying attachment theory. Hofer points out that in all mammals, including humans, the containment of the fetus within the mother's body allows maternal regulation of fetal physiology. Through the processes of placental transfer, mothers supply biologically active substances of many kinds to their babies, as well as vital blood gases, oxygen and carbon dioxide. In this way, the mother exerts physiological control of the developing fetus. There are some indications that mothers exert influence not only on fetal physiology, but also on fetal behavior. For example, on the basis of animal studies, researchers believe that pregnant

The researchers did not directly study the children's brain development. Rather, they collected detailed and comprehensive information about each child's adaptation. The study was very comprehensive, covering all major aspects of development—social, cognitive, and emotional. They looked at children's temperaments, made detailed assessments of IQ and other developmental milestones, and assessed children's language development. They also observed and assessed each child's context—including both life stresses and the ongoing social support available to them and their families.

Data collection was especially concentrated in the first two years, focusing most intensely on early attachments. The researchers paid particular attention to children's relationships with their primary caregivers, based on their conviction that children's experiences are most often filtered through those relationships.

For 180 children (and their mothers) who remained in the study through age 20, the researchers found that:

- The kinds of attachments children have formed with their primary caregivers at one year of age predict teacher ratings, behavior problems, and quality of relationships with peers in preschool. Early attachments also predict the social competency of ten- and eleven-year-olds in a summer camp setting.
- Children gain a great deal from interactions with peers over the years. Infants who experience warm, responsive caregiving are, later in life, more empathetic with peers. When they are responded to early in life, they learn something basic about what it means to be connected with other people.
- Children's development is adversely affected by numerous environmental conditions associated with poverty. The negative effects of poverty are cumulative and increase with age.
- Abuse, neglect, and trauma in the early years have a long-term, adverse effect on children's development.
- Early caregiving that is sensitive and emotionally responsive can indeed buffer the effects of high-risk environments (including maternal stress). This is especially true for boys. It can promote positive change for children who have experienced poverty and abuse, and can interrupt the transmission of abusive patterns from one generation to the next.
- By studying the early experiences of high-risk young children (from 12 to 42 months)—especially the quality of their primary attachments and the level of environmental supports—it is possible to predict children's later school achievement. The correlation was fairly strong in the first and third grades, and even stronger in the sixth grade and at age 16.
- Several factors contribute to resilience—the capacity for positive outcomes despite challenging or threatening circumstances. These factors include: emotionally responsive caregiving; early competence; a well organized home environment; well developed intellectual and language capabilities; and a low overall level of risk. The best ways to divert children from maladaptive pathways are to reduce the level of stress they experience and provide support to the family.

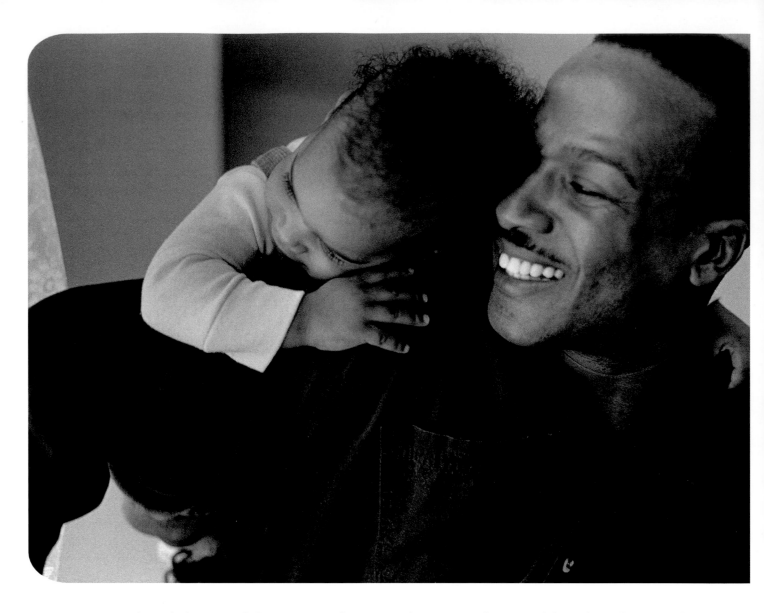

women, through their own daily activities and routines, help to set their babies' daily rhythms and sleep-wake cycles.[23]

The mother's regulatory role during pregnancy is well established. What is less well understood is the way that mothers (or other primary caregivers), by virtue of the kind of care they provide, continue to regulate babies' physiological processes *after birth*, including their neurological development. Hofer's research addresses this issue.[24] In extensive studies of rats, he has shown that a wide range of infant systems are affected or regulated by the nature of the mother-infant attachment—that is,

the nature and timing of their physical contact; the presence or absence of reciprocity in their interactions; the mother's responsiveness to the infant's own rhythms and behavioral signals; and the extent to which all of the infant's sensory systems are activated. Hofer has referred to these interactions as "hidden regulators." His studies of hidden regulators in young rats suggest that mother-infant interactions regulate many biological systems, particularly those involving reward, arousal and sleep, regulation of body temperature, and hunger. By the same token, separation from the mother has a dramatic impact on early development. Hofer's studies of rat pups show that when infants are removed from the mother two weeks after birth, dramatic physiological and biochemical effects can be observed within 24 hours, including changes in the infant's levels of growth hormone and other biologically active substances, heart rate, blood pressure, sleep patterns, sucking, and responsiveness to stimulation. Infants who are permanently separated from their mothers appear to be more vulnerable to stress later in life.

Hofer's observations rely heavily on animal studies, but he points to mounting evidence that the nature of the caregiver-infant attachment affects early human development as well. He cites, for example, studies of infants raised in chaotic or neglectful families who fail to grow at expected rates, as well as studies showing that premature infants who are touched and held on a regular basis gain weight more quickly, register greater gains in head circumference, and show greater overall improvement than those who receive less tactile stimulation.[25]

At the University of Wisconsin's Harlow Primate Laboratory, Gary W. Kraemer has illuminated the nature and impact of early attachment by studying monkeys. His research shows how neuroendocrine systems are "tuned" through caregiver-infant interactions and then carried forward. Kraemer concludes that the basic regulatory systems that shape infant behavior are acquired through interactions with a caregiver. He emphasizes the importance of interaction: this is not a one-way process. Caregivers do not simply transfer the required knowledge to young children. Rather, regulatory systems emerge out of the give and take between caregiver and infant, with the infant playing an active role. In his work with monkeys, Kraemer has also found that if the attachment process fails or the caregiver is unresponsive to the infant's needs, the infant may become socially dysfunctional. In this way, disrupted or insecure attachments can lead to problems in adulthood.[26]

Children learn in the context of important relationships.

Findings like these encourage neuroscientists to posit that hidden regulators are also present in human caregiver-infant relationships. Hofer states that some of these regulators may continue to operate in adult relationships, and that they form an important mechanism by which interaction with the environment—in this case the social environment—shapes the development of biological systems and behavior.

Based on work by Hofer, Kraemer, and others, we now have new insight into the relationship between psychology and neurobiology, and the ongoing importance of good early attachment between caregivers and infants. In addition, there is a growing body of research on children's attachments and relationships with child care providers. Recent studies show that child care does not weaken the bonds between parent and child; moreover, secure attachments to consistent child care providers—especially when providers are well trained and care for a small number of children—have been associated with better cognitive and social development, greater language proficiency, and fewer behavior problems.[27]

A final word about attachment: as we mine new knowledge about the brain to promote better results for children and their families, Maya Carlson and Felton Earls of the Harvard School of Medicine and the Harvard School of Public Health urge sustained attention not only to cognitive development, but to social development as well. The goal is not only to produce competent students and workers, but also to enhance children's capacity to become competent family members. As Earls

"Peek-boo," he says.

"Peekaboo," his father answers, spreading one big hand in front of his face and trying to get breakfast ready with the other.

"Peeka-peeka-peeka-peeka," he chants, beaming with delight.

"Peekaboo, I see you. There's my boy!"

By the time children are two, it seems easier to judge whether they are securely attached to their caregivers. You can see it in smiles that light up their eyes, in playful exchanges that celebrate a history of loving care. But as researchers seek to elaborate the role of attachment in early brain development, they must be more systematic in their approach. They need a theoretical framework that can help them explore what attachment means, how it comes about, and how it can be measured. The challenge is to bring hard science to bear on a necessarily "soft" concept.

An infant's physiology and behavior are regulated from the start by the moment-to-moment give and take between child and caregiver. Young children benefit when caregivers are able to read and respond to the signals they send. Neuroscientists can now detect the effects of a caregiver's warm, responsive care—or its absence—on the brain's biochemistry and architecture.

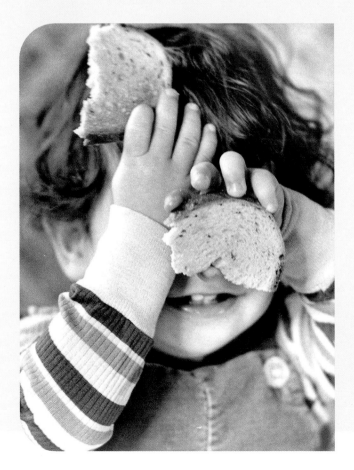

Researchers are confirming that attachment is a two-way process. This view has not always held sway. Existing scholarship on parent-child attachment springs largely from the work of John Bowlby, whose emphasis on attachment as a crucial component of early development has been immensely influential over several decades. Bowlby observed numerous babies as they interacted with their mothers. He described a control system in which babies, beginning at about six months of age, use a range of behaviors (such as smiling, babbling, crying, or visual tracking) to draw a caregiver's attention or protest separation.

In recent years, researchers have extended (and in some cases, challenged) Bowlby's theories and methods. They generally agree that babies play an active role in forming attachments, but they tend to place more weight on the regulatory role of a caregiver's sensory characteristics and behaviors.

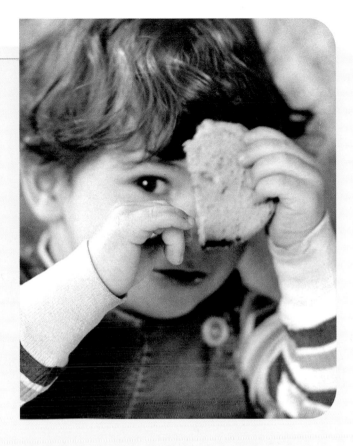

In the seventies, Mary Ainsworth and her colleagues showed that mother-child pairs differ in the quality and intensity of their attachment, and that these variations can be measured. Ainsworth devised innovative strategies for observing children, mothers, and strangers relate in a series of brief, highly structured interactions, and then gauging and classifying different types of attachment. She identified three types of children: avoidant/insecurely attached; ambivalent /insecurely attached; and securely attached.

Today, researchers tend to assess attachment with methods that require more extended, in-depth observation of children and caregivers in more natural settings. For example, the Attachment Behavior Q-Set, developed by Everett Waters and Kathleen E. Deane, of the State University of New York at Stony Brook, presents an observer with a set of cards, each containing a simple statement about a specific interaction or behavior. A card might read, for example, "When child finds something new to play with, he carries it to mother...." After several hours, the observer sorts the cards into piles that range from "most characteristic" of the child's behavior to "least characteristic."

The Q-Set method identifies three kinds of relationships that refine Ainsworth's typology. A child with a **secure** attachment exhibits specific behaviors that reflect a trusting relationship with the caregiver. A child with an **anxious/resistant** attachment is not comforted by the caregiver. When picked up, for example, she may resist by arching her back, biting, screaming, or whining. When a child has an **anxious/avoidant** attachment, she tends to behave as if the caregiver were not in the room.

Many intervention programs include home visitation, and visitors need tools that can help them assess, as objectively as possible, child-caregiver attachment. Carollee Howes of the University of California at Los Angeles has developed assessment tools for use in the Children First program, including an Adult Attachment Interview and an Adult Involvement Scale.

Intensive research into the neurobiology of attachment is now underway. Efforts to understand and measure attachment should benefit greatly from collaboration among researchers in diverse disciplines-including neuroscientists, child development experts, psychologists, and anthropologists. Collaboration should lead to new insights into children's attachments with fathers, grandparents, child care providers, and other caregivers. In addition, it promises to shed light on how attachments are formed and expressed in different cultures.

and Carlson have written, "the major social responsibility of parents (and other caretakers) is to maintain and embellish the early social concern and understanding of young children to enable them to form long-lasting relations with their own partners and children."[28]

3. | The human brain has a remarkable capacity to change, but timing is crucial. There is mounting evidence of the brain's neuroplasticity. This means that the brain has the capacity to change in important ways in response to experience. There is now ample scientific support for the view that the brain is not a static entity, and that a person's capacities are not fixed at birth. The brain itself can be altered—or helped to compensate for problems—with appropriately timed, intensive intervention. An intervention is an action, or series of actions, that parents, other caregivers, or professionals undertake in an effort to help an individual or group solve a problem, change a behavior, or improve a particular aspect of their development or functioning. Helping a mother to read her newborn's signals more accurately, reading a story to a group of toddlers, running a program that provides home visits to new parents, and performing surgery are all "interventions."

The Brain's Capacity to Compensate

Surgeons and other physicians who treat children for neurological disorders offer dramatic examples of human brain plasticity. It is well established, for example, that a child who loses language due to a stroke often recovers this capacity, because the brain transfers this function to its other hemisphere. In cases of intractable epilepsy, where it is sometimes necessary to remove an entire hemisphere of a child's brain, the remaining hemisphere generally begins to do double duty, and there can be a remarkable resurgence of vital neural pathways allowing substantial recovery of cognitive functioning.

The brain's ability to change and to recover lost functions is especially remarkable in the first decade of life. By the time children enter adolescence, recovery is certainly possible, but tends to be slower and less complete, and may require more intensive intervention. This decrease in plasticity corresponds with a drop in synapse density that accompanies the onset of puberty. But the effects are not just theoretical. Numerous case studies show that over time, the brain gradually becomes less susceptible to external influence or teaching. For example, the literature on feral children—those who have grown up without exposure to human language—suggests that they learn to speak most successfully if they are brought into contact with human society in the first decade of life.[29] The first decade is critical not only for language acquisition, but also for other cognitive functions. Visual processing also requires certain kinds of stimulation in the first decade of life. For instance, children who lose an eye before the age of eight compensate more effectively—and therefore have better depth perception—than those who lose an eye later in life. Based on new insights into brain plasticity, eye surgeons are now removing congenital cataracts much sooner, to ensure that visual acuity will not be lost.

"Prime Times" for Healthy Development

Because the brain has the capacity to change, parents and other family members, friends, child care providers, teachers, doctors, and human service providers have ample opportunities to promote and support children's healthy growth and development. Needless to say, no single strategy will

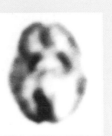

Before surgery
3 years, 11 months

Three months
after surgery
4 years, 3 months

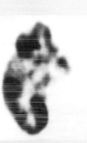

Two years
after surgery
6 years, 1 month

REMARKABLE RECOVERY: *Half of a four-year-old's brain was surgically removed to relieve the symptoms of intractable epilepsy. Within two years, the other half compensated for this loss by gaining mass and function.*
Source: H.T. Chugani

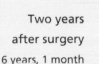

result in optimal brain development; efforts to promote children's learning must be comprehensive.

Scientists have learned that different regions of the cortex increase in size when they are exposed to stimulating conditions, and that the longer the exposure, the more they grow. Stimulation enlarges the number of dendrites in each neuron, creating larger "dendrite trees" and thickening cortical cells. Research bears out that an enriched environment

can boost the number of synapses that children form. Studies of young adults indicate about 15 percent variability in brain metabolism, which appears to correspond to the different amounts of energy needed to maintain varying numbers of synapses. Researchers believe that most of this variation reflects early experiences. [30]

People who care for children can also take heart from animal studies. William T. Greenough of the University of Illinois performed an important experiment, exposing one group of rats to a stimulating environment, and housing another comparison group in drab cages with very little stimulation. Then he looked at their brains. The rats living in an enriched environment had 25 percent more connections among their brain cells.[31] Translated into human terms, this could mean trillions of extra synapses. But the impact of an impoverished environment can be equal or even more dramatic, thinning out dendrite trees and reducing cortical thickness.[32]

More recently, research published in the April 13, 1997 issue of *Nature* showed that an enriched environment may actually increase the number of neurons in the brains of young adults. Working at the Salk Institute for Biological Studies, the researchers found that well after puberty, mice produce a modest reserve of new neurons in certain parts of their brains. The scientists suspect that experience plays a role in determining how many of these neurons survive. They found that young adult mice living in enriched settings (more complex cages with challenging objects and activities) ended up with 15 percent more neurons than those living in standard laboratory cages.

The bottom line is that the brain's plasticity presents us with immense opportunities and weighty responsibilities. But timing is crucial. While learning continues throughout the life cycle, there are "prime times" for optimal development—periods during which the brain is particularly effi-

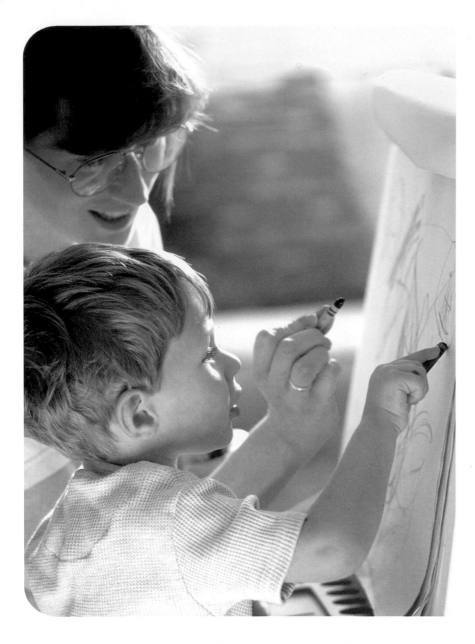

The concept of the critical period rests on the premise that neurological development depends on the exposure of the brain (and particularly the cortex) to many kinds of stimulation according to a predictable timetable. When there is a disruption of the normal developmental schedule of experience, neural connections are not made properly, and the cortical columns that result are thinner than they should be—sometimes with devastating results. For example, a normal kitten that is blindfolded during the critical period when visual stimulation is required will never have normal vision. Moreover, if that kitten receives visual input but does not get motor stimulation, this deprivation will affect the kitten's visual-motor coordination.[33]

During developmental "prime times," neurons can create synapses most easily and efficiently. This requires not only energy and sufficient neurotransmitters, but also enough synaptic space. Gary Kraemer reports, based on his studies of monkeys, that competition for synaptic space is an important feature of early brain development. For example, input from each eye competes for synaptic space in an infant's visual cortex. If one eye of an infant monkey is closed during the period when this competition takes place, the synapses formed in response to stimuli from the open eye expand into regions that would normally serve the closed eye. Even during the critical period, opening the closed eye will not restore function unless the eye that has been open is shut.[34]

cient at specific types of learning. In the neurobiological literature, these special periods are described as "critical periods" or "plastic periods." Both terms signify a span of time, in development, when significant alterations in the brain's architecture appear to be possible. As Harry Chugani observes, "Perhaps critical is not a good word. This is an opportunity, really—one of nature's provisions for us to be able to use the environmental exposure to change the anatomy of the brain and to make it more efficient." Once the prime time has passed, opportunities for forging certain kinds of neural pathways appear to diminish substantially.

It has long been known that there are optimal periods for different kinds of learning. Young children who move to a new country or community pick up the language easily, while their adolescent brothers and sisters can't shed their accents and their parents struggle to make themselves understood at all. This is not news. But now we understand that a young child can easily acquire a new language because the brain cells that process language are in the process of being wired, and are therefore especially responsive to experience.

Critical periods do not exist for brain development as a whole, but rather for each of the brain's systems. The brain's intricate circuitry is not formed at a steady pace; rather, brain development proceeds in waves, with different parts of the brain becoming active "construction sites" at different times and with different degrees of intensity. By studying the PET scans of children who came to his hospital for diagnosis and treatment, Harry Chugani and his colleagues have quantified the activity levels of different parts of the brain at various stages of development. In this way, they have gained insight into brain plasticity at particular ages. At one month of age, for example, there is intensive activity in the cortical and subcortical regions that control sensory-motor functions. Cortical activity rises sharply between the second and third months of life—a prime time for providing visual and auditory stimulation. By about eight months, the frontal cortex shows increased metabolic activity. This part of the brain is associated with the ability to regulate and express emotion, as well as to think and to plan, and it becomes the site of frenetic activity just at the moment that babies make dramatic leaps in self-regulation and strengthen their attachment to their primary caregivers. During this period, caregivers play an important role in helping infants to develop self-

regulatory capacity by responding sensitively to their emotional signals.

A final point about cortical development in infancy: the fact that increased metabolic activity in the frontal cortex coincides with rapid development of a baby's ability to form attachments and

While learning continues throughout the life cycle, there are "prime times" for optimal development— periods during which the brain is particularly efficient at specific types of learning.

self-regulate is not a simple case of cause and effect. Here again, the dynamic relationship between nature and nurture is evident. The heightened activity reflects, in part, the reinforcement of some synapses and the elimination of others, allowing complex interactions with the world; but these more complex interactions in turn lead to further reinforcement and pruning of synapses.

4. The brain's plasticity also means that there are times when negative experiences or the absence of appropriate stimulation are more likely to have serious and sustained effects. Brain development reflects a wide range of physical, cognitive and emotional experiences; the brain organizes in response to the

pattern, intensity and nature of these experience. Harry Chugani observes, "We know that rich and positive experiences stabilize certain connections in the brain." He goes on to speculate, "But what about negative experiences? What about aggression and violence? There is no reason to think that they cannot be 'stabilizing' influences in the same way. We can have individuals who, based on early experiences, are in effect 'hard-wired' for negative behaviors." Some neuroscientists consider this an overstatement; others find it too mild.

The following pages summarize presentations made at the conference on a range of major risk factors that may compromise brain development in the prenatal period and the first years of life. In each instance, there is some controversy as to the effects of particular behaviors and whether they can be distinguished from the impact of other risk factors. One further qualification: the studies cited in this section are part of a much larger literature on the impact of negative experiences on early brain development.[35] The major conclusions drawn here are supported by numerous studies of markedly different samples of children using a wide variety of research methods.

"We know that rich and positive experiences stabilize certain connections in the brain. But what about negative experiences?"

The Impact of Trauma and Neglect

Early experiences of trauma or abuse—whether in utero or after birth—can interfere with development of the subcortical and limbic areas of the brain, resulting in extreme anxiety, depression, and/or the inability to form healthy attachments to others. Adverse experiences throughout childhood can also impair cognitive abilities, resulting in processing and problem-solving styles that predispose an individual to respond with aggression or violence to stressful or frustrating situations. Researchers have shown, by observing children and their primary caregivers over time, that whether children form secure attachments hinges on the quality of care they receive; children who are abused or neglected are unlikely to be securely attached to their caregivers. The same researchers have observed, moreover, that both quality of care and security of attachment affect children's later capacity for empathy, emotional regulation, and behavioral control.[36]

But trauma or abuse are hardly the only conditions that can lead to developmental delays or impairments; as many researchers have shown, emotional neglect, social deprivation, and a chronic lack of appropriate stimulation are among the other factors that may jeopardize early development. Based on an expanded knowledge of early brain development, researchers are creating a "road map" for development—marking the key emotional milestones that children must pass at particular junctures on their way to healthy and mature development. Here again, the notion of "prime times" is important. As the brain develops in the first years of life, there are periods when children can meet a new developmental challenge most easily and efficiently. Bruce Perry of Baylor University asserts that when key experiences are minimal or absent, the result may be an inability to modulate impulsivity, immature emotional and behavioral functioning, and (in combination with other developmental experiences) a predisposition to violence.

Indeed, Perry argues that a great deal of violence in the United States today may be connected to a lack of appropriate attachments early in life. Perry suggests that violence is an outgrowth of a "malignant combination of experiences"—emotional and cognitive neglect and traumatic stress. The combined effect of neglect and trauma can lead to a dramatic impairment of the brain's capacity for modulation and regulation. When these conditions persist, the neurophysiology of the brainstem and midbrain tends to become overdeveloped. These are the areas of the brain that allow only for immediate responses related to biological survival—responses that are primitive and "hardwired," and not very susceptible to external influence.[37] Perry observes that overdevelopment of these areas is associated with anxiety, impulsivity, poor affect regulation, and hyperactivity. At the same time, cortical functions (such as problem-solving) and limbic functions (such as empathy) become underdeveloped.

The long-term research of Sroufe and his colleagues confirm the link between poor attachment and violence. The children in their study whose primary caregivers were emotionally unavailable in the early years of life did indeed exhibit (according to independent assessment) more aggression and conduct problems in childhood and adolescence.[38] Sroufe notes that across all cultures in which attachment has been studied, "anxious-avoidant attachment," which results from persistent unresponsiveness on the part of the primary caregiver, can indeed make a child more prone to violence.

Stanley Greenspan of the George Washington University School of Medicine and Health Sciences observes that children vary in their response to

Both quality of care and security of attachment affect children's later capacity for empathy, emotional regulation, and behavioral control.

neglect and trauma, based on individual differences and the organization of their particular central nervous systems. Children who are underreactive to sensations and have low muscle tone tend to respond by becoming more self-absorbed, withdrawn, passive and depressed. In contrast, children who crave sensory input and are very active are more likely to become more aggressive under these circumstances. Intense empathy and nurturing relationships along with limit-setting and practice with regulating behavior can help even the children who tend to crave sensory input become compassionate, thoughtful, and empathetic.[39]

The Impact of Maternal Depression

A number of researchers have focused their attention on specific situations in which children may not receive the warm, responsive care they need at a crucial stage of development. Some have studied the impact of maternal depression on the development of infants and toddlers.[40] A recent study by The Commonwealth Fund found that one in three birth mothers experiences symptoms of postpartum depression. Among mothers whose depression persists beyond the first six months, the symptoms come and go; but nine percent of mothers who reported lingering depression said that they experience it all of the time.[41]

When mothers' depression was treated or went into remission, their babies' brain activity returned to normal.

When postpartum depression is limited to a few months immediately after birth, it appears to have no lasting impact on children's development. But lingering depression can have adverse effects. *Starting Smart*, published by Ounce of Prevention, says, "Research has shown that parents suffering from untreated depression often fail to respond sensitively to their children's cries and bids for attention, and that they are unlikely to provide the child with the kind of cognitive stimulation that promotes healthy brain development."[42]

Geraldine Dawson and her colleagues at the University of Washington report that depressed mothers of infants tend to express less positive and more negative affect; to be less active and more disengaged from their babies; when they are engaged, tend to be more intrusive and controlling; and often fail to respond adaptively to infants' emotional signals. Their infants tend to be more withdrawn and less active than other babies. They are apt to have shorter attention spans and less motivation to master new tasks than the infants of non-depressed mothers. Dawson also reports physiological effects: infants of depressed mothers tend to have elevated heart rates and elevated cortisol levels.

Proceeding from the premise that parents' behavior shapes young children's emerging ability to express and modulate emotions, Dawson and her colleagues examined the impact of maternal depression on the biological systems involved in emotional development, especially the frontal cortex. The researchers studied the brain functions of 13-to-14-month-olds—30 children of depressed mothers and 30 children of non-depressed mothers—using EEG. The EEG was attached to babies' scalps by means of caps that use sponges and warm water as the conductive medium. This allowed researchers to conduct sophisticated brain mapping without causing the baby any discomfort whatsoever.

The researchers exposed the infants to a variety of conditions meant to elicit a variety of emotions—watching an interesting toy, playing with the mother or caregiver, or being separated from the mother. They videotaped the sessions, and correlated the videotapes with the brain mapping produced by the EEG. They found that a substantial proportion of babies with depressed mothers—about 40 percent—showed reduced brain activity. The researchers paid particular attention to the left frontal region—the part of the cortex associated with outwardly-directed emotions (such as joy, interest, or anger). Nine out of ten babies who showed high levels of left frontal activity had non-depressed mothers. On the other hand, 21 of the 28 babies who showed low levels of left frontal activity had depressed mothers.

While not all babies of depressed mothers show negative effects, the pattern is clear: maternal depression can impede healthy brain activity, particularly the part of the brain associated with the expression and regulation of emotions. Dawson is confident that the adverse effects stem primarily from the mother-child interactions, rather than from a genetic predisposition to depression. By correlating the videotapes with the EEG results, she and her colleagues found that babies showed less brain activity when their mothers were more negative and more intrusive. Furthermore, she found that in many cases, when mothers' depression was treated or went into remission, their babies' brain activity returned to normal.

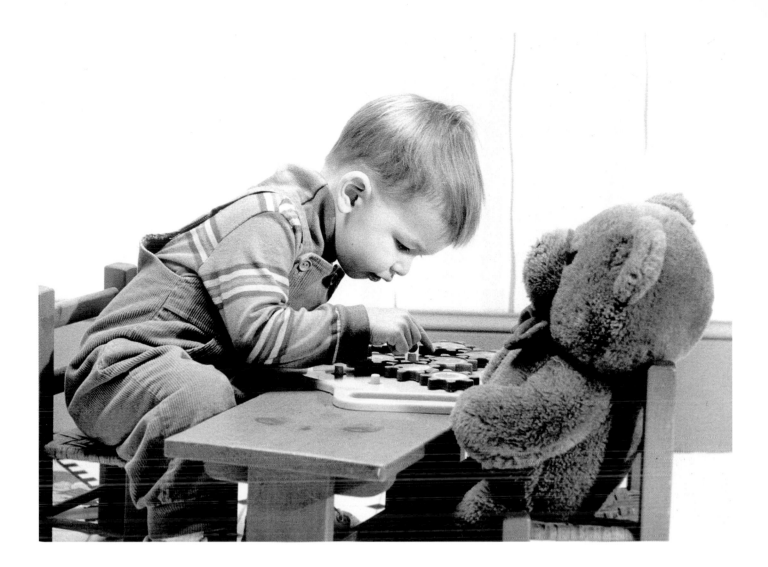

Dawson says that there is mounting evidence that the period of greatest risk for maternal depression is the period from six to eighteen months. When mothers' depression remits by the time their infants reach the age of six months, their babies do not appear to suffer later cognitive delays or emotional symptoms. In contrast, when mothers remain depressed beyond their babies' sixth month, their children tend to show later behavioral problems and cognitive impairment. As might be expected, the more persistent and prolonged a mother's depression, the more likely it is that her child will have behavioral disturbances. There is also some evidence that infants born to mothers who suffer from depression during pregnancy are less active and less responsive to social stimuli than other newborns.

This research dramatizes the need to screen for maternal depression even during the prenatal period, and the importance of encouraging mothers to seek treatment. Fathers or other family members need support as well, since a non-depressed father and a strong relationship between the baby's parents have been shown to moderate the adverse impact of maternal depression on young children.

The Impact of Substance Abuse

New knowledge about the vulnerability of the developing brain to environmental factors suggests that early exposure to nicotine, alcohol, and drugs (in utero and in the postnatal environment) may have even more powerful and long-lasting effects on young children than was previously suspected. Recent studies appear to bear this out. Most of the current research focuses on exposure to these substances during the prenatal period, although neuroscientists assume that postnatal exposure (for example, when children breathe in smoke from cigarettes or crack cocaine), also has an adverse impact on brain development.

Maternal smoking during pregnancy is associated with somewhat higher rates of preschool and school-aged behavioral problems.

Pregnant women are routinely advised by their doctors not to drink alcohol while they are planning or expecting a child, but may not know exactly why. In fact, neuroscientists are now gaining new insight into how alcohol affects prenatal brain development. Some important findings have come from animal studies. Studies of mice suggest, for example, that exposure to alcohol early in the prenatal period reduces the number of cells in the neural tube, the part of the embryo that gives rise to the brain and spinal cord.[43] Other studies have shown that when alcohol is administered to rats throughout pregnancy (5 percent alcohol in a protein-rich diet), many neurons in their babies' brains (specifically in the cortex) are smaller than expected and have fewer dendrites—parts of brain cells needed to form synapses.[44] Recent brain

research suggests that human infants who are exposed to alcohol before birth face many of the same biological consequences. For example, EEG studies have found that the brain waves of infants born to alcoholic mothers show a distinct pattern of reduced activity, particularly in the left hemisphere.[45]

Mothers who drink heavily during pregnancy are at greatest risk of giving birth to babies with fetal alcohol syndrome (FAS); some researchers believe that two or more drinks per day lead to FAS while others place the dangerous consumption level a bit higher. FAS is associated with low birthweight, later growth deficiencies, facial abnormalities, and a range of neurological disorders. Some children may show few or no adverse effects; but today, more and more children are being diagnosed with fetal alcohol syndrome. By the time they enter preschool, FAS children may show signs of mental retardation; may have impaired perceptual, linguistic, and fine motor skills; and may exhibit behavior problems.

Smoking during pregnancy can also affect early development. Estimates of the percentage of pregnant women who smoke cigarettes range from 14 to 25 percent.[46] Some of these women find it difficult to stop smoking during pregnancy, but manage to cut back. And in many cases, their children show no apparent effects. But the nicotine in tobacco products does cross the placenta and has a direct impact on the developing fetus. A number of studies indicate that maternal smoking during pregnancy can, in some cases, affect brain development, inhibiting neuron growth in particular ways. It can also alter the brain's biochemistry by affecting neurotransmitters—the chemicals that flow across synapses, allowing connectivity among brain cells. As synapses are produced, some portion of these chemicals is not needed and is therefore reabsorbed by neurons and remetabolized. Exposure to nicotine appears to interfere with the reabsorption of certain neurotransmitters, including serotonin.

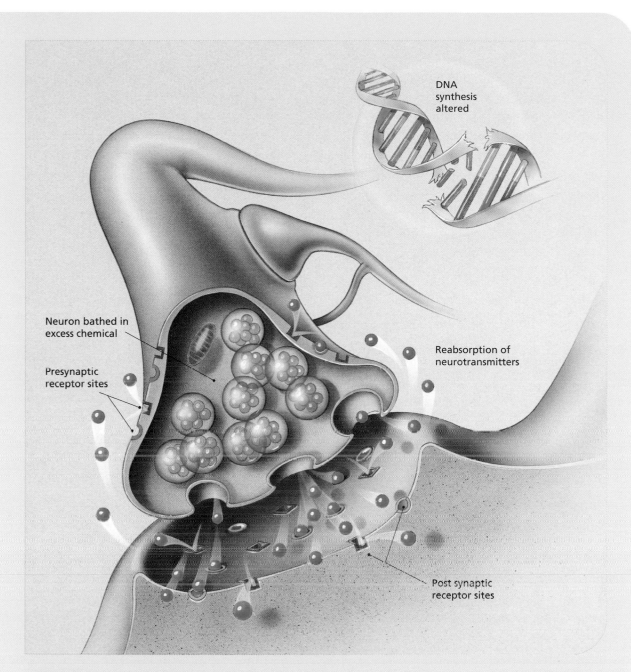

DNA synthesis altered

Neuron bathed in excess chemical

Presynaptic receptor sites

Reabsorption of neurotransmitters

Post synaptic receptor sites

HOW NICOTINE AND OTHER DRUGS MAY AFFECT SYNAPSES: When a synapse is activated, neurons release more neurotransmitters than they need and then reabsorb the excess at special receptor sites. Scientists hypothesize that drugs such as nicotine and cocaine interfere with this reabsorption by blocking receptor sites. As a result, the neurons' "connection sites" are bathed in leftover chemicals and may become overstimulated.

When that happens, scientists hypothesize, neurons are bathed in the excess chemical, increasing the level of excitation in that part of the brain. Nicotine appears to affect brain development in other ways as well. For example, animal studies suggest that exposure to nicotine can alter DNA and RNA synthesis in the brain. These changes can have clear, long-term consequences even when a fetus is exposed to levels of nicotine that are not usually considered toxic.[47]

Given these effects, one would expect children exposed to nicotine before birth to be more prone to developmental delays or impairments. And in fact, research shows that their behavior may indeed be affected. Animal studies indicate that in utero exposure to nicotine causes decreased learning efficiency and heightened motor activity. Studies of humans suggest that maternal smoking during pregnancy is associated with somewhat higher rates of preschool and school-aged behavioral problems. For example, research conducted at the University of Chicago

In the prenatal period, exposure to cocaine can interfere with the production of synapses.

showed that boys whose mothers smoke more than half a pack of cigarettes a day during pregnancy are much more likely than the sons of nonsmokers to develop conduct disorders later in life.[48]

Exposure to cocaine in utero can also be perilous. The prevalence of cocaine use among pregnant women appears to be alarmingly high. In her remarks at the conference, Linda Mayes of Yale University reported that from 17 to 50 percent of women who receive prenatal care at Yale New Haven Hospital use cocaine or crack cocaine two or three times a week throughout their pregnancies. She added that other inner-city hospitals report that as many as 50 percent of pregnant women receiving prenatal care use cocaine or crack. Mayes estimates that nationwide, at least 40,000 and perhaps as many as 375,000 infants born each year have been exposed to cocaine in utero, and often to other drugs as well. After birth, children continue

to be exposed to cocaine through passive smoke inhalation. In fact, some 17 percent of children coming to inner-city emergency rooms for clinical care test positive for exposure to cocaine.[49]

To be sure, some children who are exposed to cocaine in utero appear to suffer few ill effects; evidence of functional impairment can sometimes be hard to detect. And since expectant mothers who use cocaine often have a number of other risk factors, it is sometimes difficult to establish cause and effect. However, the research suggests that the consequences of cocaine use during pregnancy can be severe and long-lasting. Exposure to cocaine early in gestation can disrupt the migration of neurons up the cortical wall. As noted earlier, this can lead to a number of serious neurological disorders. Later in the prenatal period, exposure to cocaine can interfere with the production of synapses. To an even greater degree than exposure to nicotine, it may inhibit the reabsorption of neurotransmitters. And indeed, children exposed to cocaine in utero have been found to have disturbances in attention, information processing, learning, and memory. The physiological signs associated with prenatal exposure to cocaine include changes in children's heart rate, blood pressure, and daily cortisol cycles. Mayes' research, comparing 61 cocaine-exposed and 47 non-drug-exposed three-month-old infants, shows that exposure to cocaine tends to show up at this early age as delayed or impaired motor development.[50]

The Impact of Institutionalization

It has long been known that institutionalization has a long-lasting, adverse effect on children's social and cognitive development. Research done in the first half of this century produced solid evidence of this fact, and led to a rapid decline in the number of such institutions in the United States and Western Europe.[51] In other parts of the world, however, many children still spend their first years in large orphanages. For example, the Romanian government expanded the number of state-run orphanages in the seventies and eighties, and these places still exist despite changes in the government's maternal and child health policies.

In 1994, Maya Carlson and Felton Earls, in consultation with Megan Gunnar, went to Romania to study young children living in these institutions, where children receive adequate custodial and medical care but live in conditions that are unpredictable and make it difficult to form attachments to consistently available caregivers. Their purpose was to study the neurobiological consequences of institutionalization by measuring the children's daily cortisol levels. They also assessed the effects of social deprivation on the children's physical growth and psychological functioning. In conducting this research, Earls and Carlson were guided by the International Convention on the Rights of the Child.

The researchers found that the cortisol levels and daily cycles of the children in the orphanages were abnormal, failing to show the strong daily rhythms typical of home-reared children as young as 12 weeks of age. Compared to home-reared Romanian children of the same age, their morning cortisol levels were much lower, but became higher at noon and remained elevated into the evening hours. Depressed morning cortisol levels have been reported in children who have experienced catastrophic events, such as the Armenian earthquake of 1988, and these levels are related to symptoms of post-traumatic stress disorder.[52]

Carlson and Earls note that the social and cognitive effects of early institutionalization can be partially prevented or reversed when staff-to-child ratios are dramatically improved, when children are given the chance to form stable relationships with consistent caregivers, and when professionally

Recent advances in knowledge of young children's brains help to explain why poverty can have such a detrimental impact on early development.

staffed programs of developmental stimulation are introduced. These measures have the greatest impact if they are undertaken when children are very young. The work of other researchers has consistently shown that when children are subjected to severe psychosocial deprivation during the first two years of life, social deficits may be even more difficult to reverse than cognitive deficits.[53]

In collaboration with Megan Gunnar, Carlson and Earls are now expanding their work to include the study of adopted Romanian children.[54] Cortisol analysis is also proving useful for studying "failure to thrive" and for assessing the impact on young children of child care in various settings.[55]

The Impact of Poverty

Many of the risk factors described so far occur together, jeopardizing the development of young children and making research endeavors more challenging. Many of these risk factors are associated with or exacerbated by poverty. Indeed, recent advances in knowledge of young children's brains help to explain why poverty can have such a detrimental impact on early development.

Today, one in four American children under the age of six is growing up in poverty. The one in four figure holds as well for children under age three.[56] Given the crucial role of environmental factors in early brain development, these children are at particularly high risk of developmental delays and impairments. Economic deprivation affects the mother's and child's nutrition, access to medical care, the safety and predictability of their physical environment, the level of stress experienced by their parents and other caregivers, and the quality and continuity of their day-to-day care. Poverty also affects children's in-home and out-of-home stimulation, and their exposure to extreme stress and violence. Epidemiological surveys confirm the impact of these conditions: the risk for poor school readiness and mental retardation is highest among children from families with the lowest socioeconomic status.[57]

Research on the impact of poverty is often difficult, because it requires teasing apart the separate and independent effects of economic hardship and other related risk factors. However, a number of important studies have taken on this challenge. Alan Sroufe and his colleagues have found that

Among the protective factors that made these children more resilient, a secure attachment with their caregivers was the most important.

poverty and factors associated with poverty have a pervasively negative impact on children's functioning in several areas, and that the negative effects appear to snowball as children get older. Most of the children in their long-term study were healthy, robust babies; most were born without physical disabilities or medical problems. However, as a result of the adverse effects of poverty, most showed gradual declines in mental, motor, and socio-emotional development. Compared to low-risk children, they tended to have poor-quality relationships with their caregivers in infancy and were found to be "anxiously attached" at 12 and 18 months. Of those who attended preschool, 70 percent were considered to have difficulty getting along and cooperating with other children, regulating their emotions, and playing and functioning on their own. By the time they reached elementary school, the great majority—fully 80 percent—showed impairments serious enough to warrant some form of special education services; 18 percent were retained in the same grade sometime in elementary school.

Sroufe and his colleagues emphasize that the "decline in functioning observed at each developmental period seems to have been related to adverse living conditions, not inherent factors and traits within each child."[58] By observing infants' early environment, support, and relationships, Sroufe's team has been able to predict with reasonable accuracy later attention-deficit hyperactivity disorder (ADHD), depression, and conduct problems.

The research team also found that some children—a distinct minority—appear to thrive despite the adverse effects of poverty. In their study, two children were advanced a grade, and two were placed in classes for the gifted when they reached the sixth grade. Some children excelled in the social arena: as sixth graders, 15 percent of children in the sample were ranked by their teachers above the 90th percentile on measures of peer competence and popularity. Among the protective factors that made these children more resilient than others in the study, a secure attachment with their caregivers was the most important. In contrast, Sroufe noted that of the 44 children who were considered to be at extreme risk (by virtue of very chaotic homes or abusive caregiving relationships), none managed to thrive socially or academically.

Sroufe and his colleagues have looked beyond poverty and the general high-risk status of the families to examine factors that enabled some of these parents to care well for their children even in the face of poverty. Critical factors included knowledge of child development, social support available to the parents, and especially for parents who had been abused or neglected in their own childhood, therapy to help them resolve abuse issues. An understanding of these factors guided the development of the STEEP preventive intervention program at the University of Minnesota.[59]

5. | Substantial evidence amassed by neuroscientists and child development experts over the last decade points to the wisdom and efficacy of early intervention. There are, to be sure, some genetic disorders or neurological events (such as a massive stroke) whose consequences are difficult if not impossible to reverse, given current knowledge and methods. But study after study shows that intensive, well designed, timely intervention can improve the prospects—and the quality of life—of many children who are considered to be at risk of cognitive, social, or emotional impairment. In some cases, effective intervention can even ameliorate conditions once thought to be virtually untreatable, such as autism or mental retardation. A number of well documented studies of programs designed to help infants and toddlers and their families, such as the New Mothers Project, the

Children from families with the least formal education derive the greatest cognitive benefits from intervention programs.

Infant Health and Development Project, and the Syracuse Family Development Project, suggest that well conceived, well implemented programs can brighten children's futures. The programs cited in the following pages were designed, implemented, and/or studied by conference participants. By no means, however, do they represent the full range of initiatives and interventions that have been found to benefit young children and their families.

Addressing Social Vulnerability

Taking part in a panel discussion, Craig T. Ramey of the University of Alabama at Birmingham reported that intensive early intervention can in fact improve the cognitive developmental trajectories of socially and biologically vulnerable young children. The efficacy of early intervention has been demonstrated and replicated in diverse samples. He observed that children from families with the least formal education derive the greatest cognitive benefits from intervention programs. Moreover, the impact of early intervention appears to be long-lasting: early educational intervention is associated with an almost 50 percent reduction in the likelihood of children being held back in the same grade during the elementary years.

Ramey cited the experience of the Abecedarian Project, which he and his colleagues launched in 1972. The project involved children from 120 poor families, who were assigned to one of four groups:

Prevention and Early Intervention

Numerous efforts to support young children and their families are now underway across the nation. Many are allied with the family support movement, which is committed to the notion that to help children, we have to provide education and support to their parents as well. Many include parent education and home visits. Some of these projects have a strong research component, and have followed children over time to gauge long-term benefits. These early intervention programs take different forms, providing a range of intensive educational and support services such as home visits and high quality child care and early education. None is perfect, but on the whole they have shown significant results. Indeed, programs designed for disadvantaged children have been able to boost IQ by as much as eight points. However, without well-designed follow up services, these benefits are difficult to sustain.

The following programs are among the many initiatives designed to give infants and toddlers a good start in life. Their histories reach back 10 to 25 years, allowing researchers to draw conclusions about their long-term effects.

Carolina Abecedarian Project

From 1972 until 1985, the Carolina Abecedarian Project, an experimental study of early childhood educational intervention, provided sustained services to young children and their low-income families. This project is unique in that it served children from the first months of life through the early elementary school years. Children entered the program from six weeks to three months, and received services for the next five to eight years. Services included high quality, full-day child care for preschoolers, and regular support and education for the parents of school-age children. The infant curriculum designed especially for this program aimed to enhance cognitive, language, perceptual-motor, and social development. In the later preschool years, emphasis was placed on language development and preliteracy skills. Children also received medical treatment on site. Follow-up assessments were conducted at ages 8, 12, and 15.

The study found that:

- Young children's involvement in high quality preschool programs had positive effects on intellectual development and academic achievement.
- At age 12, participating children had IQ scores that averaged 5.3 points higher than a comparison group of non-participants.
- At age 15, compared to the comparison group, participants showed higher achievement test scores and had 50 percent fewer special education placements.

Syracuse University Family Development Project

Between 1969 and 1975, this project provided education, nutrition, health and safety, and human service resources to low-income, primarily African American, families. The services began with prenatal care and continued until children reached elementary school age. Families received home visits on a weekly basis as well as high quality child care five days a week. From 6 to 15 months, children were in half-day care; thereafter they received full-day care. The program followed children into adolescence.

The study found that:

- In grades 7 and 8, girls who had taken part in the program had higher teacher ratings and grades and better attendance records than children in the comparison group. Boys showed no long-term benefits, judging by these measures.
- Program participation decreased the total number, severity, and chronicity of later involvement with the juvenile justice system. In their teen years (ages 13-16), program participants were significantly less likely than a comparison group to have probation records or to be chronic offenders.

The Prenatal/Early Infancy Project

This rigorously evaluated early intervention program has helped young mothers improve their own health and has propelled their children on a path towards success. The Prenatal/Early Infancy Project focused exclusively on the prenatal period and the first two years of life. Beginning in 1977, this project enrolled 400 expectant mothers in Elmira, New York. Eighty-five percent were low-income, unmarried, and teenaged women expecting their first child. The full range of program services included home visits by nurses, screening for health problems, and transportation for health care. Home visits by nurses started during pregnancy and continued monthly until the child reached the age of two. They not only focused on strengthening parental caregiving, but also aimed to help mothers solve problems and plan their own futures.

By helping mothers improve their own skills, this program also helped families become economically self-sufficient. It demonstrated that comprehensive intervention early in a family's life cycle can effectively prevent some of our society's most intractable problems. Researchers who followed these 400 families from pregnancy to four years concluded that the program had more than paid for itself.

The study found that:

- Program participants had an 80 percent reduction in the rate of verified cases of neglect and abuse.
- There was an 83 percent increase in the number of years these mothers participated in the workforce.
- Reduced public assistance expenditures accounted for 80 percent of the cost savings associated with this program.

Follow-up research indicated that the program had a substantial, lifelong impact on participating families—especially for those young families facing the most extreme levels of stress. A 15-year follow-up found that participants continued to show benefits. For example, they were less likely to rely on welfare. For children born into low-income households where mothers were unmarried, there was more than a 50 percent reduction in the rates of abuse and neglect.

Continues on next page

The Infant Health and Development Program

The Infant Health and Development Program (IHDP) provided services to low-birth-weight, premature infants and their families from birth to age three. Established at eight sites serving diverse populations, IHDP began operating in 1984. The program provided home visits over the three-year span, center-based child care with an educational curriculum focused on child development, and group meetings for parents with children between one and three years of age. The children also received regular pediatric care. Compared with low-birth-weight, premature children who received only pediatric care, the IHDP children showed substantial gains.

The study found that:

- At age three, program participants had significantly higher mean IQ scores. Heavier infants scored 13 IQ points higher than infants receiving only pediatric care. Lighter infants scored almost seven IQ points higher than infants receiving less comprehensive services.
- IHDP program participants also had fewer cognitive, behavioral and health problems.
- At age eight, the heavier group continued to register modest gains in their cognitive and academic skills.

the first group received intensive early education in a child care center from about four months of age to age eight; the second group, from four months to age five; the third, from age five to age eight; and the fourth group received no intensive early education services. The early intervention program provided a range of services including early childhood education, family counseling and home visits, health and nutrition services, social work and service coordination services, speech/language services, and transportation. Many of these components were forerunners of those services now specified under Part H (birth to three years) of the Individuals with Disabilities Education Act. Ramey stresses that nothing was done in the Abecedarian program that could not, with sufficient planning and effort, be incorporated into other preschool centers or school systems.

This study showed that the earlier the children received intensive care and education, the greater and more enduring the gains. In fact, children who did not begin receiving the intervention until after the age of five showed no gains in academic performance or IQ. A follow-up study concluded that intellectual and academic gains attributable to the program persisted through seven years in school. In fact, the difference between the intensive early intervention and control groups was more pronounced at age 12 than at age 8.

Ramey also presented findings from two other early educational intervention programs designed to prevent mental retardation and improve school readiness and educational progress. Data from Project CARE (a successor to the Abecedarian Project) show that children who received a full-day, five day per week center-based program supplemented by home visits showed much higher intellectual performance than those who received home visits only or those in a control group who received no services.

The Infant Health and Development Program (IHDP) extended the aims of the first two programs, showing that lower birthweight children benefit less from the same high quality intervention program than other children, probably due to their biological status. It also established a correlation between the level of family participation and the extent to which children benefitted from the program. The more the family participated, the greater the cognitive gains.

Developmental Care for Preterm Infants

All human babies are born with brains that are remarkably unfinished—rough drafts waiting for life's rewrites and edits. The fact that the brain is a work in progress means that from the first days of life, the impact of early experience can be dramatic. This is especially true for preterm infants, who come into the world with brains that have had less time to mature in the protected intrauterine environment, and are therefore even more vulnerable to the environment.

In this vulnerable condition, most preterm babies have been cared for in neonatal intensive care units (ICUs)—settings that have traditionally been designed to meet their medical rather than their developmental needs. In this bright, noisy, rather stark setting, preterm infants have been exposed to severe sensory overload—a dramatic mismatch with the needs and expectations of their nervous systems.[60] Moreover, many preterm babies have been deprived, for sustained time periods, of three environments that have been shown to support healthy development: the protective environment of the uterus; the comfort and tactile stimulation of a parent's embrace; and containment in a family's social group. In her presentation, Linda Gilkerson, reporting on her research and the work of Heidelise Als of Harvard University and others, stated that developmentally appropriate and sup-

portive care for preterm infants—care that is relationship-based and family-centered—can substantially increase preterm infants' chances for physical and mental health, while reducing hospital stays and costs. Gilkerson and her colleagues have researched the impact of such care. In a study of 38 randomly selected preterm infants who weighed on average less than two pounds, 20 were able to leave the hospital after an average of 87 days as compared to an average 151 days for the 18 infants in the control group. Hospital costs for the care of these 38 infants dropped by approximately $90,000, compared with average expenditures in a traditional neonatal ICU. Research has also shown that while heavier preterm infants respond most dramatically to enhanced care, those who are at highest risk of poor outcomes—those born with very low birth weights and multiple medical complications—also show improvement in their medical and developmental status when they receive intensive, individualized developmental care.

Preterm infants come into the world with brains that have had less time to mature in the protected intrauterine environment, and are therefore even more vulnerable to the environment.

Gilkerson described the Newborn Individualized Developmental Care and Assessment Program (NIDCAP), a model developed as a framework for providing developmental care to preterm infants. This model trains hospital personnel to observe the behavior of every infant and then develop an individualized caregiving plan based on his or her unique characteristics, particularly the baby's sleep-wake cycles and self-soothing strategies. Parents play a fundamental role in this process and in the delivery of care. The neonatal ICU has been redesigned to provide a greater sense of security,

Researchers can detect auditory processing problems in babies six to nine months old that usually lead to language impairment.

protection, and intimacy through the frequent presence of parents, a great deal of physical contact and containment by parents and caregivers, attention to the pacing of care, and continuity of care providers. They use low lights, reduce noise, and, whenever possible, schedule doctors' rounds to accommodate the babies' sleep cycles. Preterm infants cared for in this setting have shown improved patterns of brain functioning, particularly in the frontal lobe which plays a crucial role in the executive functions of the brain such as attention state regulation and planning.

Brain Research and Neurological Impairments

New insights into the brain's early development and functioning have allowed some researchers to design interventions that address neurological impairments with greater precision. The research cited below offers examples.

Stanley Greenspan's work with autistic children poses two key questions: Can the environment be designed to help children overcome central nervous system differences—including both those that are hard-wired at an early age, and those that remain plastic and flexible? To what extent is it possible to help children recover function or learn new functions for the first time? Based on his experience working with children with a range of different developmental delays or impairments, Greenspan has concluded that children's capacity to respond to intervention in the early years is "greater than we thought."

Greenspan presented the case of a boy diagnosed with autistic spectrum disorder who first came to his attention a few months before his third birthday. His behavior was characterized by repetitive actions: he would repeat the alphabet in a mechanical way, and would spend a lot of time lining up objects. At other times he seemed aimless; occasionally, he would produce an appropriate sound, word, or gesture. Greenspan began an intensive program encompassing family support, speech work, occupational therapy, and an interactive play approach called "floor time." This approach is designed to take into account a child's particular central nervous system patterns and expressions, as well as his or her current developmental level. It rests on the concept that not all experiences, however stimulating, will help the central nervous system grow and recover functions. Rather, specifically designed experiences are necessary to help children with impairments develop new capacities. This work has also led to the identification of specific types of experiences that can facilitate both intellectual and emotional growth in children without impairments as well.

Over time, the boy presented by Greenspan became more interactive, creative, and more socially adept. He began to form gratifying friendships, and his IQ went up to a high range. By age eight, he was highly verbal, fully conversational, warm, engaging, and creative. He enjoyed friendships and was doing well in a challenging academic program in a regular school. In all, Greenspan and his colleagues have worked with about 200 children diagnosed with autistic spectrum disorder, and he reports that about two-thirds of these children have responded well to his program, challenging the notion that they will inevitably be limited, socially and cognitively, as adults.[61]

To be sure, not every autistic child benefits to the same degree from this kind of program. Citing the research of Michael Rutter, Alan Sroufe notes that children who do not have language and those with tested IQs below 50 do not usually respond well to intervention.[62] Sroufe believes that success stories should be presented carefully, so that they do not inspire false hope in parents with autistic children.

A second example of an intervention that has emerged from recent brain research is the work that April Benasich and her colleagues at Rutgers University are doing with infants and toddlers who have auditory processing problems. They have designed early interventions for children who have a specific language impairment—a developmental speech or language disorder that cannot be traced to any known cause. Benasich reports that from 3 to 10 percent of preschool children have been found to have this type of disorder.[63]

With the aid of brain imaging studies, the Rutgers researchers have concluded that these children's problems can often be traced to a faulty brain mechanism which existed well before language problems became apparent to parents or pediatricians. Benasich and her colleagues can detect auditory processing problems in babies six to nine months old that usually lead to language impairment. The ability to assess these processing problems in the first year of life, in conjunction with a more general assessment of an infant's perceptual-cognitive abilities, is an important step towards early intervention for children at high risk for language-based learning disabilities. Once a problem has been pinpointed, specific, individualized interventions can be introduced at a time when the brain's plasticity is particularly marked. For example, by means of specially designed computer games, children can be taught to speed up the rate at which they process shifts, within words or phrases, from one sound to another.

Information gathered by neuroscientists about the sequence and timing of brain development can be immensely useful to parents, teachers, health providers, policy makers in diverse fields, and other people responsible for the well-being of children and families. What kinds of learning experiences (including toys and games) are appropriate for children of different ages? What is the right age to begin reading instruction? When children appear to have difficulty with a particular cognitive task, what is the best time to intervene? When and how should children be given opportunities to begin learning foreign languages? Insight into developmental prime times can shed light on questions like these. The concluding section of this report addresses the policy questions that new knowledge about the brain most frequently elicits.

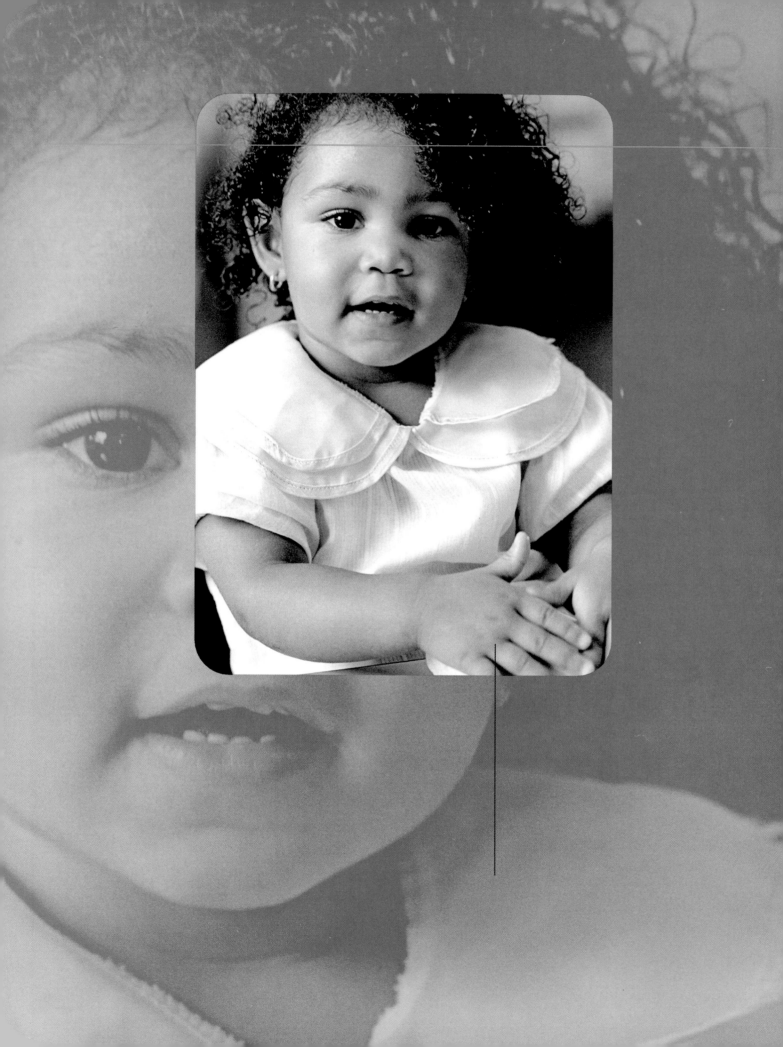

Where Do We *Go From Here?*

Nobel Laureate Murray Gell-Mann opened his remarks to participants at the June 1996 brain conference by observing that in most spheres of knowledge, what we don't know far exceeds what we do know. Brain research is no exception. Coming years promise to yield new discoveries about how the brain develops and how children's capacities grow and mature. Neuroscientists are likely to shift their attention from more general questions about how brain circuitry is formed to more specific investigations of the functions of particular regions of the brain. This investigation is also likely to focus on how—and how much—the brain's development and functioning are influenced by the environment.

Where is the Consensus?

There appeared to be substantial agreement among speakers at the conference that the current knowledge base is sufficiently ample to warrant immediate action. A framework for action, speakers agreed, might be designed around key assertions summarized in this report, including the importance of the interplay between nature and nurture; the importance of secure early attachments; the extent and rapidity of early development; the brain's remarkable plasticity; and the wisdom and efficacy of prevention and high-quality well-designed early intervention.

During the discussions, three key principles of societal responsibility emerged that appeared to have resonance for most participants:

■ **First, do no harm.** The evidence is clear and compelling: early and developmentally appropriate care and education are vital to the health and well-being of our children. The prenatal period and the first three years of life are particularly crucial. As Edward Zigler of Yale University underscored, new insights into the brain suggest that the principle that guides medical practice should be applied just as rigorously to all policies and practices that affect children: first, do no harm.

This means enabling parents to fulfill their all-important role in providing and arranging for sensitive, predictable, reliable care for their children. Research on the impact of early attachments on brain development confirms that warm, responsive caregiving is a crucial ingredient in the healthy development of children. But unless parents have consistent access to a wide range of services—including (but not limited to) prenatal care and adequate nutrition; competent, responsive care during and following childbirth; affordable parental leave; and high-quality, affordable child care and health care—efforts to improve results for

In most spheres of knowledge, what we don't know far exceeds what we do know. Brain research is no exception.

Who is a Caregiver?

Child Care and Early Education

When reports about young children are written, it is always a struggle to find a word or phrase to describe the grownups who take care of them. Mothers? Yes, but not always. Parents? That takes fathers into account, but what about Grandpa or Aunt Martha? And what about the neighbor who "watches" the twins five days a week while mom and dad are at work? Or Ms. Sanders, the teacher at the Rainbow Child Care Center?

To be sure, a "child care provider" can play an immense role in children's early development. But that term doesn't do justice to parents and other people who have primary responsibility for a child. And so, we have resorted to "caregiver." Often we speak of the "primary caregiver"—the adult who has major responsibility for a child's day-to-day well-being and development. It's a word that can apply to mothers or fathers or Grandma or Ms. Sanders.

Of course, it is awkward to use one word for such different kinds of relationships, but that awkwardness may have an advantage. It points up the important idea that relatives and child care providers do not replace working parents. They may relate to a child differently than a mother or father would, but from a child's perspective, every important caregiver is a potential source of love and learning, comfort and stimulation. From a neuroscientist's perspective, every important caregiver has the potential to help shape a young child's future.

Child Care/Early Education Demand and Supply

The number of mothers with infants and toddlers who work outside the home has surged in recent decades. In l965, 21 percent were in the labor force; by 1994 that number reached 59 percent. This dramatic increase has created an unprecedented demand for child care services. The growing number of working mothers is not the only reason for this rise in demand. A third of all families in which the mother does not work outside of the home also use a regular child care arrangement for their youngest preschool-age child.

To meet this demand, the supply of child care has risen sharply. In 1990, there were 80,000 centers in the United States, serving between four and five million children. In addition, it is estimated that there are 118,000 regulated homes serving 700,000 children. There are also approximately 685,000 to 1.2 million family child care homes that are not licensed or registered, serving 3.4 million children.

Despite this increase, there appear to be gaps between supply and demand. This problem is especially acute for infants and toddlers. Moreover, parents are hard pressed to find child care that is affordable and meets their quality standards. In a nationally representative study of the U.S. workforce, 58 percent of parents looking for child care reported that they found no realistic options in their communities.

A Shift in Child Care Settings

Over the past 25 years, the arrangements that families rely on to care for their children have shifted. There has been a sharp drop in the use of care by relatives other than parents, such as grandparents, aunts, and uncles. Among families with employed mothers of infants and toddlers, 36 percent arrange for care in the homes of friends, neighbors, relatives, or regulated family child care providers; 23 percent use centers. Preschool children average 35 hours in their primary arrangement if their mothers work outside of the home, and 20 if they do not. Infants who are in center-based care spend more hours each week in child care than older children.

Child Care Quality

Mounting concern about the quality of child care across the nation reflects a growing consciousness that for many children, child care is "education before school." A recent report, based on a three-year study known as Quality 2000, asserts that the U.S. is now facing a "quality crisis" in early care and education.

There is ample evidence for this assertion. Three multi-site observational studies of both center care and family child care conducted between 1988 and 1994 reveal a dismal picture of quality. These studies indicate that only 12 to 14 percent of children are in child care arrangements that promote their growth and learning; at the same time, from 12 to 21 percent are in child care arrangements that are unsafe and jeopardize their development. The statistic for infants and toddlers is even more alarming: 35 to 40 percent spend their days in settings that have been deemed detrimental to their health, safety, and development.

The hallmark of quality for non-parental care is not very different from quality of care by mothers or fathers: warm, responsive, consistent caregiving geared to the needs of individual children. Researchers have identified specific, interrelated characteristics of center-based settings associated with high-quality early care and education and better results for children. These include:

- a sufficient number of adults for each child—that is, high staff-to-child ratios;
- smaller group sizes;
- higher levels of staff education and specialized training;
- low staff turnover and administrative stability; and
- higher levels of staff compensation.

The capacity of providers to offer responsive care on a consistent basis hinges, in part, on what goes on "behind the scenes"—the laws, regulations, funding, licensing and training that create a context for quality. In particular, quality is affected by state regulations. Children who live in states with high regulatory standards have higher quality early care and education than children who live in states with low standards.

Continues on next page

In family child care (care in the home of the provider), children fare better emotionally and cognitively when their caregivers:

■ are committed to taking care of children and are doing so from a sense that this work is important and it is what they want to be doing;

■ seek out opportunities to learn about children's development and child care, have higher levels of education, and participate in family child care training;

■ think ahead about what the children are going to do and plan experiences for them;

■ seek out the company of others who are providing care;

■ are regulated by the states;

■ have slightly larger groups (three to six children) and slightly higher numbers of adults per child; and

■ charge higher rates and follow standard business and safety practices.

As in center-based arrangements, studies find that these characteristics of quality go together. Providers who have one of these characteristics are likely to have others. In other words, providers who are intentional in their approach provide more sensitive and responsive education and care.

Improving Quality

There are indications that the quality of care and early education is declining. Although the educational level of staff has improved, ratios and group sizes appear to be getting worse. Furthermore, numerous programs do not meet their own state standards for group size and staff-to-child ratios, especially in programs for infants and toddlers. Compensation remains low, and not surprisingly, staff turnover is high.

Recent studies encourage some optimism about efforts to improve quality. A study of family child care training by the Families and Work Institute revealed that children are more likely to be securely attached to providers who have received effective training, and that the quality of the caregiving environments has improved somewhat. Another study by the Families and Work Institute showed that when the state legislates higher staff-to-child ratios and more rigorous educational requirements for staff, children clearly benefit: they are more securely attached, exhibit better cognitive and social development, are more proficient with language, and have fewer behavior problems.

children will have to keep their focus on after-the-fact intervention rather than on prevention or promotion. Policies or practices that prevent parents from forming secure attachments with their infants in the first months of life require urgent attention and reform. At the same time, parents need more information about how the kind of care they provide affects their children's capacities; they also need reassurance that there are many ways to meet children's needs, and that learning to read their infants' and toddlers' cues is one of the most important ways they can promote healthy brain development.

"First, do no harm" also means mounting intensive efforts to improve the quality of child care and early education, so that parents can be sure that when they are at work, their young children's learning and emotional development are being fostered. Today, more than half of all mothers with babies under the age of one work outside of the home. Most American children of preschool age attend some type of out-of-home child care. And the vast majority of them spend their days in settings that have been judged by researchers to be of mediocre to poor quality. Infants and toddlers receive lower-quality care, on average, than three- or four-year-olds. Now that neuroscientists have documented the impact of early experience on our youngest children, and now that we know beyond a doubt that adverse conditions can dramatically impair their functioning, it is no longer reasonable to wait until children are five to worry about the quality of their care and education.

■ Prevention is most effective, but when a child needs help, intervene quickly and intensively. Knowing that early experience has such a decisive influence on brain development, parents may worry that every unpleasant sensation or upsetting experience will become a neurological nightmare. They may rest assured that in most cases, a history of consistent and responsive care cushions children from the ups and downs that are inevitable in everyday life; in fact, minor mishaps are among the stimuli that promote healthy development and help children cope with stress later in life. Given timely and intensive help, children can scale a wide range of developmental hurdles; moreover, they can often recover even from serious stress or trauma.

The brain is, after all, a work in progress, designed to be adjusted and fine tuned throughout life. Certainly there are conditions that cannot be significantly remedied or repaired, given today's knowledge. But the list of conditions that can be prevented or improved is growing, as researchers and practitioners learn more about what works (and why) for diverse children with diverse needs.

There is widespread agreement about the value of early intervention, but to have the greatest impact it must be timely and well-designed, and it must be followed up with appropriate, sustained services and support. In coming years, more detailed knowledge about specific aspects of brain

Risk is not destiny. The medical, psychological, and educational literatures contain a sufficient number of examples of people who develop or recover significant capacities after critical periods have passed to sustain hope for every individual.

development and functioning will allow the design of interventions that more closely match children's needs, and that can be offered at the time when they can do the most good.

■ Promote the healthy development and learning of every child. There was wide agreement among speakers at the conference that children who do not receive appropriate nurturing or stimulation during developmental prime times are at heightened risk for developmental delays or impairments. There was also general agreement that if we miss early opportunities to

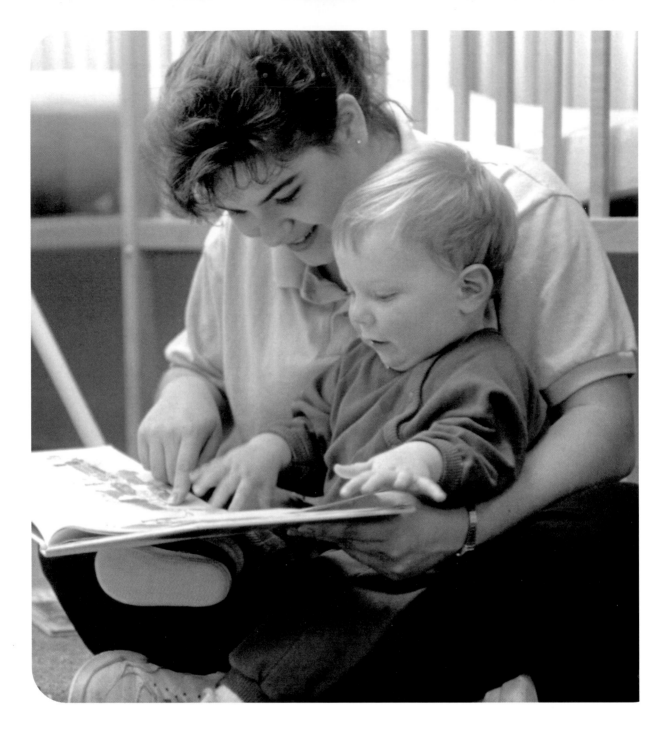

promote healthy development, later remediation may be more difficult and costly, as well as less effective, given the knowledge, methods and settings that are currently available.

However, this theme was sounded repeatedly: *risk is not destiny*. Numerous cases were cited of individuals who have thrived despite adverse conditions. The medical, psychological, and education-

al literatures contain a sufficient number of examples of people who develop or recover significant capacities after critical periods have passed to sustain hope for *every* individual. Ongoing efforts to enhance cognitive, emotional, and social development must be supported in every phase of the life cycle.

Where Is the Debate?

Presentations and discussions at the conference not only revealed new insights into early brain development; they also highlighted issues that have sparked controversy. Disagreements—about substance or emphasis—clustered about three related questions. Each points to possible directions for future research.

■ **Which plays a greater role in early brain development—nature or nurture?** Today, most experts on early development, whether neurobiologists or psychologists, tend to view brain development as a dynamic process, described by Stanley Greenspan as "an elaborate dance between biology and the environment."[64] But which partner leads and when? Is it the genetic endowment that most severely limits an individual's capacities? Or is it the environment? These questions continue to spark controversy wherever brain development is discussed.

■ **Is the brain flexible throughout the early years, or only at certain times?** This debate focuses on the question: just how critical are critical periods? Neuroscientists have established that there are time spans when different parts or systems of the brain are more or less vulnerable to environmental influence. But how long are these critical periods? And when they draw to an end, do windows of opportunity (and risk) slam shut? Or are they merely lowered?

Some neuroscientists acknowledge the brain's unique plasticity, but emphasize that the developing brain—particularly the cortex—requires specific stimuli on a fairly rigid schedule. For example, Bruce Perry has written that during critical periods, "specific sensory experience is required for optimal organization and development of any brain area... Absent such experience and develop-

ment, dysfunction is inevitable...."[65] Writing about the development of sensorimotor systems in primates, Gary Kraemer describes "neural patterns that will not exist unless the organism has certain experiences and makes certain responses to them....[S]ensory mechanisms can be tuned, but at some point their functional characteristics must be 'locked.'" Kraemer adds that the "locking process itself may occur even if expected stimuli have not arrived. Thereafter, sensorimotor systems cannot be tuned to the environment the way they would have been at an earlier developmental stage."[66]

Others argue that in most areas of early development, "prime times" stretch for rather extended periods. For example, Harry Chugani notes that until about age 12, the human brain can, with relative ease, master many cognitive functions that adolescents and adults learn with more difficulty, such as acquiring languages or learning to play a musical instrument.

This debate also touches on the brain's capacity to repair itself. Is this capacity limited to very brief periods? Studies of spontaneous recovery by individuals who have suffered brain damage tend to support the notion of rather brief prime times during which neuroplasticity allows the brain to repair itself. However, other neuroscientists stress that we do not yet understand the brain mechanisms responsible for spontaneous recovery. New research on spinal cord injuries suggests that, to a greater extent than scientists previously thought, regional reorganization can occur in adulthood.[67]

■ **Given what we know about the impact of early experience on brain development, should we broaden our understanding of "resilience"?** It is often assumed that in all but extreme cases, children can bounce back from the hurts and disappointments that life inevitably brings. Indeed,

Tough Questions

New insights into early development point to this conclusion: the experiences children have and the attachments they form in the first three years of life have a decisive, irrefutable impact on their later development and learning. As more and more evidence emerges supporting this finding, parents, teachers, and policy makers are beginning to pose tough questions. A full discussion of these issues is beyond the scope of this report; the following paragraphs merely frame four key questions, and suggest directions that the search for solutions might take.

■ Should new mothers stay home?

Since warm, responsive care is so crucial in the first years of life, shouldn't mothers or fathers put off going back to work and devote all of their time to caring for their infants and toddlers? This longstanding debate may be rekindled as the relationship between secure attachment and healthy brain development is better understood. It is a reasonable question, so long as the decision remains a personal, family matter, and so long as working parents are not blamed for any and every developmental hurdle their children encounter. Given the economic realities of their lives, millions of women do not have the option of staying home, even in their child's first year. Today, most working women (55 percent) are indispensable providers, contributing half or more of family income. New welfare requirements compel many others to work or attend training programs. Moreover, research shows that deep-seated guilt and anxiety about balancing work and family can harm not only mothers, but also children; when mothers believe that they are doing the wrong thing, either by working or by staying at home, children may be adversely affected. Research also shows that high quality care can enhance a child's development. Ultimately, what is best for families is to have real choices, and that requires policies and societal attitudes that support parents whether or not they work outside the home. In particular, families need access to affordable, high quality child care and early education.

■ What should be done when parents do not provide their children with the kind of care and setting that promote healthy development?

This wrenching issue has been the subject of heated debate in recent years, and promises to stir more controversy in the future. Americans appear to be particularly concerned about young children being raised by teenaged parents. Some have proposed placing young children from chaotic, neglectful, or abusive homes in orphanages, but this approach makes no sense in view of research showing the adverse impact of institutionalization on brain development. Others have suggested foster care for young mothers *and* their children. How can parents be helped and, when appropriate, supervised effectively, so that families can stay together? How can existing parent education efforts and family support programs be strengthened or extended? The challenge in coming years will be to search for answers that support both families and young children.

■ Can we realistically hold out hope for children whose early development is compromised?

This is not an academic question. How it is answered affects the expectations parents and teachers convey to children; the placements and tracking decisions made by school administrators and teachers; and the kinds of decisions judges and juries hand down when juvenile offenders stand before them. As a society, we should never give up on any child. To be sure, as children move into the second decade of life, it appears to be more difficult to bring about change, but it is not impossible. As researchers learn more about brain plasticity, new ways to promote the development of people of all ages are likely to emerge. Moreover, brain development is not just a matter of intellectual development, but also physical, emotional, and social well-being. Children whose development is delayed in one area may have extraordinary capacities in other spheres that are less apparent and less likely to be measured.

■ Should we withdraw resources from older children and give them to young children?

How should we, as a nation, invest in the next generation, given the importance of early development? Should public education begin sooner and end earlier? If so, which agencies or organizations should provide that early education? Should we fund high schools at lower levels, in order to devote adequate resources to child care and early education? The relationship between budgets and policies is always complex, and there is no simple solution. But ensuring children's healthy development is not a zero-sum game. To be sure, good nutrition is vital in the prenatal period and the first years of life, but the needs of young children cannot justify skimping on the nourishment provided to older children and youth. By the same token, the early years are certainly crucial for healthy development, but there must also be strong support for school-age children and adolescents, as well as for adults who want to continue their education and strengthen their skills. Optimal development and learning for Americans of all ages must be a top national priority, so that a good start in life for our youngest children is not purchased at the expense of their older brothers and sisters.

scholars have produced numerous studies of resilience, showing that it resides not solely in the child, but also in the context in which he or she lives. This research reports that children who grow up in deprived or disadvantaged settings can adjust well to the demands of school and become successful learners if they have access to a supportive community and a strong bond with at least one adult whom they can count on in their extended family or neighborhood.[68]

But given new findings about how early experiences—both positive and negative—affect brain development, our current understanding of resilience may not be sufficiently broad or complex. Reliable support from a coach or an aunt may certainly help to buoy children's self-esteem and strengthen their survival skills. And a supportive community network certainly can make a difference. But we need to know much more about a wide range of protective factors—biological, psychological, social, and ecological—that affect an individual's ability throughout life to withstand stress and to thrive despite all odds.

Implications for Policy and Practice

New insights into early development confront policy makers and practitioners in many fields with thorny questions and difficult choices. Some of these questions deal with communicating new findings and engaging the public in efforts to promote healthy development. How can we convey to parents, caregivers, and teachers the opportunities and risks of the early years of life without creating paralyzing anxiety, or without setting off a frenzy of inappropriate or ill-considered enrichment efforts? How can we emphasize the opportunities of the early years without dimming hope or shrinking resources for adolescents and adults?

Mothers and fathers are not—and must not be made to feel—solely responsible for every hurdle their children may encounter.

Other questions reflect the dilemmas that confront policy makers in every sphere of human services. How do we balance support for universal policies and programs, designed to achieve optimal development for all children, with support for initiatives that focus on those children who live in settings or conditions most likely to jeopardize healthy brain development? How can we scale up national initiatives that address the needs of our youngest children, such as Early Head Start, while allowing for flexibility and initiative at the state and local levels? What can we learn from other countries that have launched promising efforts to reduce risks to early brain development?

There needs to be a lively, sustained national debate about the health and well-being of America's children. As we move into the next century, our children need and deserve policies that reflect the importance of the early years, and that reflect the principles that emerged from the brain conference.

In particular, new knowledge about early development adds weight and urgency to the following policy goals identified in several major reports.[69]

■ | Improve health and protection by providing preventive and primary health care coverage for expectant and new parents and their young children. Expectant mothers and fathers must have access to the care, knowledge, and tools they need to protect their babies. The prenatal period is a time of active brain development. And yet, one in five pregnant women receives little or no prenatal care in the crucial first trimester; for African American, Latina, and American Indian women, the number is one in three. In addition to prenatal care, pregnant women need safe homes, adequate nutrition, and buffering from extreme stress. With adequate health care and parenting supports, there is a great deal that expectant mothers and fathers can do to promote the healthy development of their children, and to avoid serious risks.

The first three years of life are also filled with important health and safety risks, but millions of children in this age span are uninsured or underinsured. Basic medical care should focus on young children's physical and emotional health and well-being. It should include preventive health screening, well-baby care, timely immunization, and information and supports for parents. This kind of care is cost-effective and provides a sturdy foundation for a lifetime of good health.

■ | Promote responsible parenthood by expanding proven approaches. All parents can benefit from solid information and support as they raise their children; some need more intensive assistance. There is solid evidence that effective parent education/family support pro-

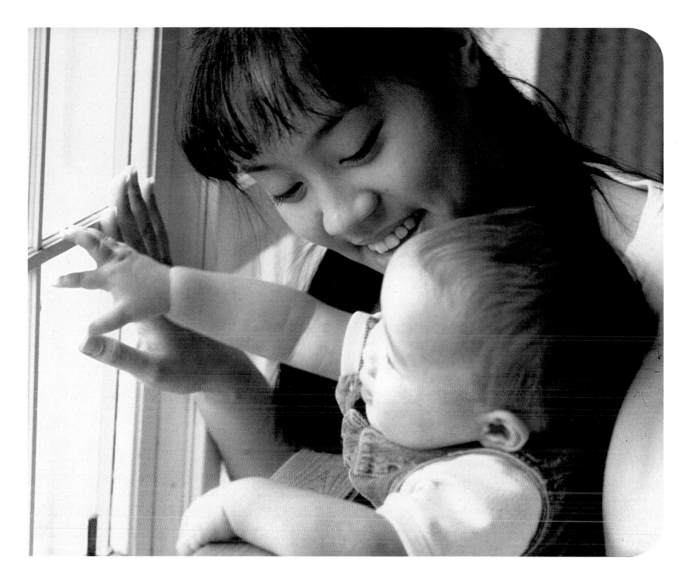

grams promote the healthy development of children, improve the well-being of parents, and are cost-effective.

■ Safeguard children in child care from harm and promote their learning and development. Researchers have found that most child care settings are of mediocre to inadequate quality, and the nation's youngest children are the most likely to be in unsafe, poor quality child care. More than one–third are in situations that are detrimental to their development. Most of the rest are in settings where very little learning is taking place. In effect, we are warehousing millions of children during their most formative years. The "first, do no harm" principle applies powerfully to early care and education. Studies show that it is possible to improve quality, creating settings in which children can thrive and learn. This is a large task, but even modest changes can make a difference: for example, a national study of family child care found that after providers received 18 to 36 hours of training, children were more likely to be securely attached to them and the quality of caregiving environments improved.[70]

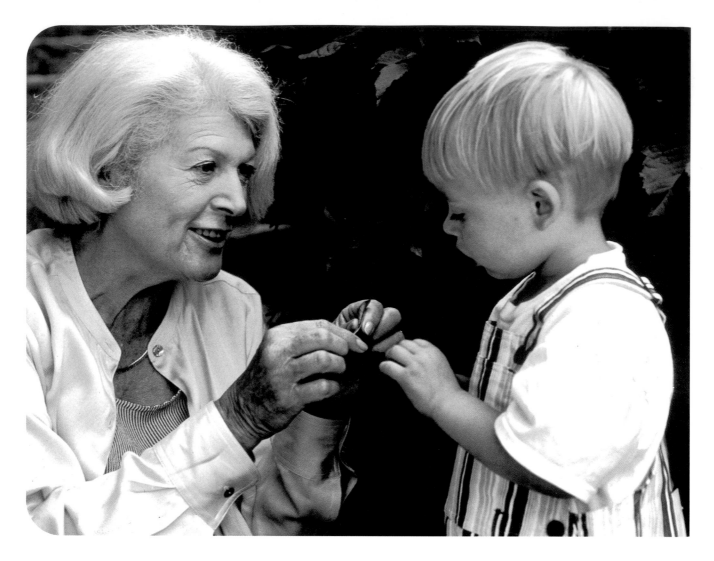

■ Enable communities to have the
flexibility and the resources they
need to mobilize on behalf of
young children and their families.

Piecemeal programs appear to be less effective than
programs embedded in comprehensive efforts to
rebuild communities. A grassroots effort is now
underway across the nation to mobilize on behalf
of young children and their families—to bring
together decision makers, to create a vision of the
kind of community they want to be part of, to
develop goals and sustainable strategies for achiev-
ing that vision, to determine how to finance their

efforts, and to make provisions for gauging
results.[71] These efforts should be carefully studied
and further developed. They need and deserve support from national, state, and local leaders, as well
as from leaders of business, the media, community
organizations, and religious institutions.

Conveying New Knowledge about the Brain

Finally, new knowledge about the brain must be
communicated to families and the public at large
with immense care. While parents have a powerful
impact on their children's development and learning, many factors play a role; mothers and fathers

are not—and must not be made to feel—solely responsible for every hurdle their children may encounter. While warm, responsive care does indeed help to promote healthy development, some neurological conditions remain fairly resistant to change. And while the neuroscientist's lens may appear to magnify or isolate such neurological problems, they are in fact only one facet of these children's rich and complex lives. The notion of critical periods also needs to be carefully qualified. To be sure, nature provides prime times for development and learning, but parents and other caregivers can take advantage of these times in many ways, drawing upon their own varied resources and beliefs. Moreover, it is never too late to improve the quality of a child's life.

In short, new insights into early brain development suggest that as we care for children in the first years of life, and as we institute policies or practices that affect their day-to-day experience, the stakes are very high. The research tells us that the "quiet crisis" of America's youngest children may have even more serious, lasting consequences for children and families, and for the nation as a whole, than we previously realized. But we can draw strength from the knowledge that there are many ways that we as parents, as caregivers, as citizens, and as policy makers can address this crisis. We can take comfort in the recognition that there are many ways to raise healthy, happy, smart children. We can take heart in the knowledge that there are many things that we as a nation can do, starting now, to brighten their future and ours.

Glossary

AMYGDALA. An almond-shaped mass of gray matter located in each half of the cerebrum near the hippocampus. Part of the limbic system, the amygdala is concerned with the expression and regulation of emotion and motivation.

ATTENTION–DEFICIT DISORDER. See ATTENTION–DEFICIT HYPERACTIVITY DISORDER.

ATTENTION–DEFICIT HYPERACTIVITY DISORDER (ADHD). A syndrome of learning and behavioral problems that is characterized by difficulty in sustaining attention, by impulsive behavior, and often by excessive activity.

AUTISM. A disorder originating in infancy that is characterized by a limited ability to interact socially, stereotyped ritualistic behavior, and language dysfunction.

AXON. The part of a neuron (brain cell) that carries outgoing signals to another neuron. A neuron usually has only one axon.

BRAIN SCAN. A computerized image of the brain produced by brain imaging technologies. See MAGNETIC RESONANCE TECHNOLOGY (MRI) AND POSITRON EMISSION TOMOGRAPHY (PET).

CELL MIGRATION. The movement of a cortical neuron during development to its proper position on the cortical wall.

CEREBELLUM. A large component of the brain situated between the brainstem and the back of the cerebrum. It is concerned with maintaining the body's equilibrium and coordinating movement. The cerebellum relays signals to the muscles from higher brain regions where decisions are made. Recent studies indicate that it also plays an important role in cognitive functions.

CEREBRAL CORTEX. The neuron-rich, furrowed, outer portion of the cerebrum. The cortex controls higher mental functions, such as thinking, planning, remembering, and analyzing.

CEREBRUM. The large, rounded structure of the brain that includes the cortex. The cerebrum controls and integrates motor, sensory, and higher mental functions including thought, reason, emotion, and memory. It is divided into two hemispheres that are joined by the corpus callosum.

CORTEX. See CEREBRAL CORTEX.

CORTICAL LADDERS. A phrase often used to describe long glial cells in the cortex. For normal development to occur, neurons must climb these cortical ladders at the right time, and must reach the right destinations.

CORTICAL NEURON. A brain cell that is located in the cerebral cortex.

CRITICAL PERIOD. A time span when a particular part of the brain is most apt to change and most vulnerable to environmental influences.

DENDRITE. A hairlike structure within a neuron that receives incoming signals from another neuron. Each neuron has many dendrites.

DENDRITIC TREE. A network that forms as the number of dendrites in a neuron multiplies. The growth of dendritic trees explains, in part, why individual neurons get bigger and heavier as the brain develops.

ELECTROENCEPHALOGRAPH (EEG). An instrument that detects and graphs the brain's electrical activity in the form of waves.

GLIAL CELLS. The brain contains two main kinds of cells—neurons and glial cells. Glial cells support and complement the various functions of neurons. In the cerebral cortex, long glial cells form "cortical ladders" that neurons must climb to reach their proper positions during brain development. This process is known as neuronal migration or cortical cell migration.

HEMISPHERE, RIGHT AND LEFT. The two halves of the cerebrum.

HIPPOCAMPUS. A curved elongated ridge that is an important part of the limbic system. It has been shown to play an important role in organizing memories.

HYPERACTIVITY. A state of being excessively active.

HYPOTHALAMUS. The part of the brain that lies below the thalamus. Its functions include regulating body temperature, certain metabolic processes, and other autonomic activities.

LIMBIC SYSTEM. A group of cortical and subcortical structures (including the cingulate cortex, the hypothalamus, the hippocampus, and the amygdala) that are especially concerned with emotion and motivation.

MAGNETIC RESONANCE IMAGING (MRI). A medical technology that produces computerized images of tissues and organs using magnetic energy.

NEURAL PATHWAY. A series of synapses that forms a network in the brain. These pathways can be activated by a particular experience.

NEURON. A cell that is part of the brain or central nervous system. Each neuron contains an axon, a cell body, and numerous dendrites.

NEURONAL MIGRATION. See CELL MIGRATION.

NEUROPLASTICITY. The capacity of the brain to change or adapt in response either to experience or to damage.

NEUROTRANSMITTERS. Chemical substances, such as serotonin or dopamine, that enable electrical impulses to pass across a synapse from one neuron to another.

PLASTICITY. See NEUROPLASTICITY.

POSITRON EMISSION TOMOGRAPHY (PET). A brain imaging technology that generates a computerized image not only of the brain's structure, but also of activity levels in various parts of the brain.

PRUNING. A term often used to describe an important feature of brain development—the selective elimination of synapses.

SYNAPSE. A connection between two brain cells, formed when the axon of one neuron hooks up with the dendrite of another neuron.

THALAMUS. The thalamus is the brain's "relay station" because it receives input from the body's sensory, motor, and other systems and dispatches them to the appropriate region of the cerebral cortex.

ULTRASOUND. The use of ultrasonic waves for diagnostic or therapeutic purposes, usually to visualize an internal body structure or monitor a developing fetus.

VESICLE. A small sac, usually containing fluid. In a neuron, vesicles are containers for neurotransmitters.

Appendix A

Conference Speakers, Respondents and Moderators

April Ann Benasich, PhD
Assistant Professor of Neuroscience
    and Director of Infancy Studies
Center for Molecular and
    Behavioral Neuroscience
Rutgers University

Barbara T. Bowman, MA
President
Erikson Institute

Marie M. Bristol, PhD
Health Scientist Administrator
NICHD/NIH

Bettye Caldwell, PhD
Professor of Pediatrics
Pediatrics/CARE
Arkansas Children's Hospital

Gaston Caperton
Former Governor
State of West Virginia

P. Lindsay Chase-Lansdale, PhD
Associate Professor
The Irving B. Harris Graduate
    School of Public Policy Studies
The University of Chicago

Maria D. Chavez, PhD
Senior Program Director
Family Development Program
University of New Mexico

Harry Chugani, MD
Director, PET Center
Children's Hospital of Michigan
Professor of Pediatrics, Neurology
    and Radiology and Director of
    Epilepsy Surgery Program
Wayne State University
    School of Medicine

Donald J. Cohen, MD
Director
Yale Child Study Center

Geraldine Dawson, PhD
Professor of Psychology
Department of Psychology
University of Washington

Felton Earls, MD
Professor of Human Behavior and
    Development
Department of Maternal and
    Child Health
Harvard School of Public Health

Emily Fenichel, MSW
Associate Director
ZERO TO THREE

Ellen Galinsky, MS
President
Families and Work Institute

James Garbarino, PhD
Director
Family Life Development Center
Cornell University

Murray Gell-Mann, PhD
Director
John D. & Catherine T. MacArthur
    Foundation

Linda Gilkerson, PhD
Director
Irving B. Harris Infant Studies
    Program
Erikson Institute

Nick Goodban
Vice President of Philanthropy
McCormick Tribune Foundation

Stanley I. Greenspan, MD
Clinical Professor of Psychiatry
    and Behavioral Sciences and
    Pediatrics
George Washington University
    Medical School

Irving B. Harris
Chairman
The Harris Foundation

Myron A. Hofer, MD
Professor of Psychiatry
Director, Division of
    Developmental Psychobiology
Columbia University College of
    Physicians and Surgeons
New York State Psychiatric
    Institute

Jeffrey P. Jacobs
Founder, Civitas Initiative
President, Harpo Entertainment
    Group

Rachel Jones
National Correspondent
Knight-Ridder, Inc.

Woodie Kessel, MD
Director
Division of Science, Education
    and Analysis
Maternal and Child Health Bureau
Health Resources and Services
    Administration
Department of Health and Human
    Services

Ronald Kotulak
Science Writer
Chicago Tribune

J. Ronald Lally, EdD
Director, Center for Child &
    Family Studies
WESTED/Far West Laboratory

Bennett L. Leventhal, MD
Professor of Psychiatry & Pediatrics
Chairman (Interim)
Department of Psychiatry
Director of Child and Adolescent
    Psychiatry
The University of Chicago

Michael H. Levine, PhD
Program Officer
Carnegie Corporation of New York

Alicia F. Lieberman, PhD
Professor of Medical Psychology
University of California San
    Francisco
Infant-Parent Program
San Francisco General Hospital

Margaret E. Mahoney
President
MEM Associates, Inc.

Linda C. Mayes, MD
Arnold Gesell Associate Professor
    of Child Development
Pediatrics and Psychology
Yale University Child Study Center

Harriet Meyer, MA
Executive Director
The Ounce of Prevention Fund

Judith Musick, PhD
Author

Bruce D. Perry, MD, PhD
Director, Civitas Child Trauma
    Programs
Baylor College of Medicine

Kyle D. Pruett, MD
Clinical Professor of Psychiatry
Yale Child Study Center

Pasko Rakic, MD, ScD
Professor and Chairman
Section of Neurobiology
Yale University School of Medicine

Craig T. Ramey, PhD
Co-Director
Civitan International Research
    Center
University of Alabama at
    Birmingham

Edward L. Schor, MD
Medical Director
Iowa Department of Public Health

The Reverend Dr. Kenneth B.
    Smith
President
The Chicago Theological Seminary

L. Alan Sroufe, PhD
William Harris Professor of
    Child Psychology
Institute of Child Development
University of Minnesota

Roger Weissberg, PhD
Professor of Psychology
The University of Illinois at
    Chicago

Bernice Weissbourd, MA
President
Family Focus

Edward Zigler, PhD
Sterling Professor of Psychology
Director of the Bush Center
Yale University

Appendix B

Examples of Early Intervention Programs

Program Name	Program Description	Study Description Program Costs Program Funding	Cost Savings	Other Impacts
High/Scope Perry Preschool Project Ypsilanti, MI	Three- and four–year-old children attended a preschool program 5 days per week, for 2.5 hours per day. The preschool program was comprehensive, including education, health and family support services.	A total of 133 children were randomly assigned to either a program group or a comparison group. Since the study's inception in 1963, researchers have been tracking a variety of indicators, including: utilization of special education services, juvenile delinquency and arrests, teen pregnancy, employment history, and post-secondary education. The latest report followed both the program group and comparison group through 27 years of age. Two years of the program cost $14,400 per child. It was funded by the state of Michigan.	By the time participants reached age 27, every $1 invested in the program had yielded savings of $7.16 in costs that might have been incurred if the program had not existed. The program savings to taxpayers (in constant 1992 dollars discounted annually at 3 percent) is estimated to be $88,433 per child from the following sources: ■ savings in schooling, due primarily to reduced need for special education services. ■ higher taxes paid by preschool program participants because they had higher earnings once they entered the work force. ■ savings in welfare assistance ■ savings of the criminal justice system and to potential victims of crimes. **Bottom Line:** The economic return from the Perry Preschool program outperformed the stock market from 1963-1993.	The follow-up study of participants at age 27 showed that program group members were more likely than the comparison group to: ■ report monthly earnings of $2,000 or more (29% versus 7%). ■ Own their own homes (36% versus 13%). ■ Own second cars (30% versus 13%). Other key findings included: ■ Program group members were less likely than comparison group members to receive welfare assistance or other social services (59% versus 80%).

Source:
Schweinhart, L.J., H.V. Barnes, and D.P. Weikart. 1993 *Significant benefits: The High/Scope Perry Preschool Study Through Age 27.* Monographs of the High/Scope Educational Research Foundation, No. 10. Ypsilanti, MI: High/Scope Press.

Program Name	Program Description	Study Description Program Costs Program Funding	Cost Savings	Other Impacts
Carolina Abecedarian Project Chapel Hill, NC	Children between the ages of 6 weeks and 5 years received early childhood education 5 days a week, year round. The parents of children between the ages of 5 and 8 were in a parent involvement program.	A total of 111 children were randomly assigned to either a comparison or program group. There were 3 different program groups — educational services, preschool program only and primary school program only. Services cost approximately $10,000 per student per year. Funding was from public education dollars from federal, state and local governments.	An investment of $10,000 per year for one child can yield an estimated minimum savings to society of approximately $100,000 per child. (This number may understate actual savings realized.) The savings reflect reduced spending on special education, welfare and juvenile crime.	Services begun during children's preschool years had positive impacts on their intellectual development and academic achievement At age 12: ■ children in the program group had IQ scores that measured 5.3 points higher than those in the comparison groups. At age 15: ■ children who participated in the preschool years earned significantly higher scores in both reading and math. ■ overall 31.2% of members in the program group were retained in grades compared to 54.5% of members in the comparison group. ■ 24% of the children in the program group utilized special education services, contrasted with 48% of the children in the comparison group.

Sources:
Campbell, F.A. C.T. Ramey. 1994. *Effects of Early Intervention on Intellectual and Academic Achievement: A Follow-Up Study of Children from Low-Income Families.* Child Development. 65:684-698.

Campbell, F.A., and C.T. Ramey. 1995. *Cognitive and School Outcomes for High-Risk African-American Students at Middle Adolescence: Positive Effects of Early Intervention.* American Educational Research Journal. 32(4):743-772.

Program Name	Program Description	Study Description Program Costs Program Funding	Cost Savings	Other Impacts
Parents as Teachers (PAT) St. Louis, Missouri	Parents with children from birth to age five received information on child development through home visits, parent groups, and referrals for needed services that the program could not offer. Their children received periodic health screenings.	This evaluation studied a sample of 400 families in 37 diverse school districts across the state of Missouri. These families were randomly assigned to a program group or a comparison group. The evaluation looked at intellectual and language abilities of children at age 3 and improvements in parents' knowledge of child development and childrearing practices.

Funding sources: Local, state, and federal funding streams and private sources including foundations, hospitals, churches, and businesses.

Average annual cost per family to provide Parent as Teachers Service: $646. | Cost savings data are not available for the study of the Missouri program. In some Parents as Teachers programs, where cost savings have been calculated, special education costs have been drastically reduced for developmentally delayed children who participated in the program.

For example, one small study of a Texas Parents as Teachers program showed that 45 percent of children were delayed in some area of development upon entry into the program. However, upon completion, researchers found that 75% of the developmentally delayed children no longer needed special services and were able to participate in a regular classroom setting.

The average cost for a child to attend a regular classroom in this Texas community is nearly $5,000 per year, compared to $12,500 per year for special education. This reveals a $7,500 cost savings when special education is averted. | In the Missouri study:
■ At age 3, Parents as Teachers children performed significantly higher than national norms on measures of intellectual and language abilities.
■ Most children from minority families did better than average on performance measures of achievement and language abilities.
■ A follow-up study which re-evaluated the children when they were in first grade, found that compared with other first-graders, 55% of PAT children were rated "above average" by their teachers. Teachers also reported that 74% of PAT parents *always* assisted with homework. |

Sources:
Pfannenstiel, J., T. Lambson, V. Yarnell. 1991. *Second Wave Study of the Parents as Teachers Program.* St. Louis: Parents as Teachers National Center, Inc.

Pfannenstiel, J., T. Lambson, V. Yarnell. 1996. *The Parents as Teachers Program: Longitudinal Follow-Up to the Second Wave Study.* Oakland Pk, KS: Research and Training Associates, Inc.

Program Name	Program Description	Study Description Program Costs Program Funding	Cost Savings	Other Impacts
Prenatal/ Early Infancy Project Elmira, NY	Home visits by nurses started during pregnancy and continued on a monthly basis until the child was 2 years old. This home visitation program aimed to improve: ■ outcomes of pregnancy (i.e. reduction in low-birthweight and preterm babies). ■ qualities of parental caregiving (including reducing associated child health and development problems). ■ maternal life course development (helping women return to school, find work and plan future pregnancies).	The study sample included 400 program participants in a semi-rural community in Elmira, NY. Of these participants, 85% were low-income, unmarried and teenaged young women who were pregnant with their first child. Participants were randomly assigned to one of three groups: the first received home visits by nurses; the second received home visits plus transportation for health care and screening for health problems; the third received only transportation and screening. In 1980, the program cost $3,173 per family for 2.5 years of intervention. (In 1996 dollars, the program costs were estimated to be $7,800 per family.) Funding sources: federal, state and local government dollars.	The initial investment in this program ($3,173) was recovered with an added dividend of about $180 (1980 dollars) per family within two years after the program ended. Additional studies on the long-term benefits of this program are now underway in Elmira, New York, Memphis, Tennessee; and Denver, Colorado. The savings reflect decreased spending on welfare and food stamps; increased tax revenues because of a higher labor force participation rate; and a reduction in costs related to child abuse and neglect. Specifically, research shows that reduced Medicaid, welfare and food stamp expenditures accounted for 80% of cost savings.	Results demonstrated: ■ Among women who smoked, those who were visited by nurses had 75% fewer preterm deliveries. ■ Among young adolescents (aged 14-16 year), those who were visited by nurses had babies who were nearly 400 grams heavier that those in the comparison group. During the first two years after delivery: ■ Program participants had a 15% lower incidence of reported neglect or abuse. ■ Program participants paid 87% fewer visits to the physicians for injuries and poisoning after the program ended. ■ Program participants lived in homes with fewer safety hazards; and their homes were more conducive to a child's intellectual and emotional development. ■ Four years after the birth of their first children participants had 42% fewer second pregnancies and 83% of mothers had jobs. 15 years later: ■ Program participants used welfare 2.5 years less ■ They had fewer subsequent children. ■ For children born into households where mothers were unmarried and low-income, there was more than a 50% reduction in the rates of abuse and neglect. ■ There were 67% fewer arrests for these mothers.

Source:
Olds, D.1997 The Prenatal/Early Infancy Project. In George W. Albee & Thomas. Gullotta, *Editors. Primary Prevention Works,* Vol. VI of Issues in Children and Families' Lives. Thousand Oaks, CA:Sage Publications, pp.41-67.

Program Name	Program Description	Study Description Program Costs Program Funding	Cost Savings	Other Impacts
The Infant Health and Development Program	Infants at eight sites received pediatric follow-up, a developmentally-focused early care and education program, and family support. Major goals: reducing developmental and health problems among low-birth-weight, premature infants.	The evaluation was designed to assess the efficacy of combining early child development and family support services with pediatric follow-up. A total of 985 infants, stratified by site and weight, were randomly assigned to one of two groups. The first group received, through age three, pediatric follow-up as well as an early care and education program focused on child development, and family support. The comparison group received only pediatric follow-up.	A formal cost/benefit analysis has not been a part of this study.	■ At age three, the program group had significantly higher mean IQ scores than the comparison group. ■ Heavier infants in the program group scored 13.2 IQ points higher than the lighter infants in the comparison group. ■ Lighter infants in the program group scored 6.6 IQ points higher than lighter infants in the the comparison group. ■ Children in the program group exhibited fewer behavioral problems than children in the comparison group.

Source:
Brooks-Gunn, J., F. Liaw, and P. Klebanov. 1992. *Effects of Early Intervention on Cognitive Function of Low Birth Weight Preterm Infants.* Journal of Pediatrics: 120:350-9.

Program Name	Program Description	Study Description Program Costs Program Funding	Cost Savings	Other Impacts
Avance Parent Child Education Program San Antonio, Texas	Children from birth through age two received educational child care (3 hours per week) while parents attended three-hour classes for the first year of the program. Parents could also participate in adult literacy programs and English as a second language (ESL) classes. Participants were high-risk, low-income families. Most were Mexican American. The major goal: to help the families develop strong parenting skills.	At each of two sites, mothers were divided into two groups: a program group and a comparison group. Mothers in the comparison groups did not receive any services during the course of the evaluation. All groups were followed for two years from the time they enrolled. Mothers were evaluated at the end of the first year and again one year later to assess changes in parenting knowledge and interactions with their children. Services cost approximately $1,616 per family per year. Funding sources: federal, state and local governments as well as private sources including foundation and corporate giving.	Although a cost/benefit analysis has not been performed for this initiative, the results in the next column demonstrate that the program has had a positive impact on mothers' behaviors.	Compared with mothers in the comparison groups, mothers in the program: ■ Provided a richer, more educationally stimulating environment for their children —a factor that has been linked to later academic success. ■ Were more active in verbally communicating with and teaching their children. ■ Talked more to their children and initiated more playful interaction with them.

Source:
Walker, T.B., G.G. Rodriguez, D.L. Johnson, and C.P. Cortez. 1995. Avance Parent-Child Education Program. In S. Smith and I..E. Sigel, Editors, *Advances in Applied Developmental Psychology: Vol. 9. Two Generation Programs for Families in Poverty: A New Intervention Strategy*. Norwood, NJ: Ablex, p.67-90.

Notes

1. Cost, Quality, and Child Outcomes Study Team. 1995. *Cost, Quality, and Child Outcomes in Child Care Centers.* Denver, CO: Department of Economics University of Colorado at Denver;
Galinsky, E., C. Howes, S. Kontos, and M. Shinn. 1994. *The Study of Children in Family Child Care and Relative Care.* New York: Families and Work Institute.
Kagan, S. L. and N. E. Cohen. 1997. *Solving the Quality Problem: A Vision for America's Early Care and Education System.* New Haven: Yale University.

2. Boyer, E. L. 1991. *Ready to Learn: A Mandate for the Nation.* Princeton: Carnegie Foundation for the Advancement of Teaching, p. 7.

3. Ramey, C. T. and S. L. Ramey. 1996. *Prevention of Intellectual Disabilities: Early Interventions to Improve Cognitive Development.* Birmingham: University of Alabama Civitan International Research Center.

4. Alexander, K. L. and D. R. Entwisle. 1988. Achievement in the first 2 years of school: Patterns and processes. *Monographs of the Society for Research in Child Development* 53(2):1;
Bloom, B. B. 1964. *Stability and Change in Human Characteristics.* New York: Wiley;
Carnegie Task Force on Learning in the Primary Grades. 1996. *Years of Promise: A Comprehensive Learning Strategy for America's Children.* New York: Carnegie Corporation of New York;
Entwisle, D. R. and K. L. Alexander. 1993. Entry into school: The beginning school transition and educational stratification in the United States. *Annual Review of Sociology* 19:417;
Krause, P. E. 1973. *Yesterday's Children.* New York: Wiley;
Lloyd, D. N. 1978. Prediction of school failure from third-grade data. *Educational and Psychological Measurement* 38 (4) 1193–1200.

5. Teo, A., E. Carlson, P. J. Mathieu, B. Egeland, and L. A. Sroufe. 1996. A prospective longitudinal study of psychosocial predictors of achievement. *Journal of School Psychology* 34 (3):285-306.

6. Carnegie Task Force on Learning in the Primary Grades. 1996. *Years of Promise: A Comprehensive Learning Strategy for America's Children.* New York: Carnegie Corporation of New York;
Rossi, R. and A. Montgomery, eds. 1994. *Education Reforms and Students at Risk: A Review of the Current State of the Art.* Washington, DC: U. S. Education Department, American Institutes for Research; Chapter 7 focuses on the tension between the importance of early intervention and the role of remedial and special education approaches. For a summary of the literature on the impact of early intervention on literacy, see Siegel, D. F. and R. A. Hanson. 1992. Prescription for literacy: Providing critical educational experiences. *ERIC Digest.* Bloomington: ERIC Clearinghouse on Reading and Communication Skills.

7. Greenspan, S. I. 1997. A developmental approach to intelligence. Abstracted from Greenspan, S. I. with B. L. Benderly. 1997. *The Growth of the Mind and the Endangered Origins of Intelligence.* Reading, MA: Addison Wesley.

8. For a discussion of the interplay between temperament and the environment, see Martin, R. P. 1994. Child temperament and common problems in schooling: Hypotheses about causal connections. *Journal of School Psychology* 32:119-134. See also:
Angleitner, A. and J. Strelau, eds. 1994. *Explorations in Temperament: International Perspectives on Theory and Measurement.* New York: Plenum;
Galinsky, E. and David, J. 1988. *The Preschool Years: Family Strategies that Work—From Experts and Parents.* New York: Ballantine Books.
Halverson, C.F. Jr., G.A. Kohnstamm, R. P. Martin, eds. 1994. *The Developing Structure of Temperament and Personality from Infancy to Adulthood.* Hillsdale, NJ: Lawrence Erlbaum Associates;
Prior, M. 1992. Childhood temperament. *Journal of Child Psychology and Psychiatry* 33:249-279;
Teglasi, H. Assessment of temperament. 1995. *ERIC Digest.* ERIC Clearinghouse on Counseling and Student Services, Greensboro NC.

9. Huttenlocher, P. R. 1984. Synapse elimination and plasticity in developing human cerebral cortex. *American Journal of Mental Deficiency* 88:488-496.

10. Chugani, H. T. 1997. Neuroimaging of developmental non-linearity and developmental pathologies. In R. W. Thatcher, G. R. Lyon, J. Rumsey, and N. Krasnegor, eds. *Developmental Neuroimaging: Mapping the Development of Brain and Behavior.* San Diego: Academic Press, pp. 187-195.

11. Chugani, H. T. 1997. Neuroimaging of developmental non-linearity and developmental pathologies. In R. W. Thatcher, G. R. Lyon, J. Rumsey, and N. Krasnegor, eds. *Developmental Neuroimaging: Mapping the Development of Brain and Behavior.* San Diego: Academic Press, pp. 187-195.

12. Remarks by H. T. Chugani. 1996. Conference: Brain Development In Young Children: New Frontiers for Research, Policy and Practice. University of Chicago, June 13-14.

13. Rakic, P. 1988. Specification of cerebral cortical areas. *Science* 241 (July 8):170-176.

14. Rakic, P., J.-P. Bourgeois, and P. S. Goldman-Rakic. 1994. Synaptic development of the cerebral cortex: Implications for learning, memory, and mental illness. In J. van Pelt, M. A. Corna, H. B. M. Uylings and P. H. Lopes da Silva, eds. *The Self-Organizing Brain: From Growth Cones to Functional Networks.* Elsevier Science BV.

15. Shore, B. 1996. *Culture in Mind: Cognition, Culture, and the Problem of Meaning.* New York: Oxford University Press, p. 3.

16. Remarks by M. A. Hofer. 1996. Conference: Brain Development In Young Children: New Frontiers for Research, Policy and Practice. University of Chicago, June 13-14. For a synthesis of the research on language acquisition, including a discussion of prenatal experience and language learning, see J. L. Lock. 1993. *The Child's Path to Spoken Language:* Cambridge: Harvard University Press.

17. Dawson, G., D. Hessl, and K. Frey. 1994. Social influences on early developing biological and behavioral systems related to risk for affective disorder. In *Development and Psychopathology.* Cambridge: Cambridge University Press, pp. 759-779.

18. Gunnar, M. R. 1996. Quality of care and the buffering of stress physiology: Its potential in protecting the developing human brain. University of Minnesota Institute of Child Development.

19. Egeland, B., E. Carlson, and L. A. Sroufe. 1993. Resilience as process. *In Development and Psychopathology.* Cambridge: Cambridge University Press; L. A. Sroufe, B. Egeland, and T. Kreutzer. 1990. The fate of early experience following developmental change: Longitudinal approaches to individual adaptation in childhood. *Child Development* 61:1363-1373.

20. Perry, B. D. 1996. Incubated in terror: Neuro-developmental factors in the "cycle of violence." In J. D. Osofsky, ed. *Children, Youth and Violence: Searching for Solutions.* New York: Guilford Press.

21. Erickson, M. F., J. Korfmacher, and B. Egeland. 1992. Attachments past and present: Implications for therapeutic intervention with mother-infant dyads. In *Development and Psychopathology.* New York: Cambridge University Press, pp. 495-507.

22. Lieberman, A. F. and C. H. Zeanah. 1995. Disorders of attachment in infancy. *Infant Psychiatry* 4(3):571-587.

23. Hofer, M. A. 1988. On the nature and function of prenatal behavior. In W. Smotherman and S. Robinson, eds. *Behavior of the Fetus.* Caldwell, NJ: Telford Press.

24. Hofer, M. A. 1995. Hidden regulators: Implications for a new understanding of attachment, separation, and loss. In S. Goldberg, R. Muir and J. Kerr, eds. *Attachment Theory: Social Developmental and Clinical Perspectives.* Hillsdale, NJ: The Analytic Press.

25. See Frank, D. A., P. E. Klass, F. Earls, and L. Eisenberg. 1996. Infants and young children in orphanages: One view from pediatrics and child psychiatry. *Pediatrics* 97 (April): 571; Als, H. and L. Gilkerson. 1995. Developmentally supportive care in the neonatal intensive care unit. *Zero to Three* (June/July):2-9; Als, H., G. Lawhon, F. H. Duffy, G. B. McAnulty, R. Gibes-Grossman, and J. G. Blickman. 1994. Individualized developmental care for the very low-birth-weight preterm infant: Medical and neurofunctional effects. *Journal of the American Medical Association.* 272 (September 21):853-891.

26. Kraemer, G. W. 1992. A psychobiological theory of attachment. *Behavioral and Brain Sciences* 15(3):511.

27. Howes, C., E. Smith, and E. Galinsky. 1994. *The Florida Child Care Quality Improvement Study: Interim Report.* New York: Families and Work Institute; Howes, C. and C. E. Hamilton. 1993. Child care for young children. In B. Spodek, ed. *Handbook of Research on the Education of Young Children.* New York: Macmillan, pp. 322-336. Howes and Hamilton report that children "are able to form secure or positive relationships with teachers even if they have insecure attachment relationships with their mothers. The relationship with the teacher may compensate for an insecure relationship with the parents. The troubling note is that teachers, though they are significant people in children's lives, are not stable." (p. 330).

28. Earls, F. and M. Carlson. 1993. Towards sustainable development for American families. *Daedalus* 122:93-121.

29. Curtiss, S. 1981. Feral children. In J. Wortis, ed. *Mental Retardation and Developmental Disabilities XII.* New York: Brunner Maisel.

30. Remarks by H. T. Chugani. 1996. Conference: Brain Development In Young Children: New Frontiers for Research, Policy and Practice. University of Chicago, June 13-14.

31. Greenough, W. T., J. E. Black, and C. Wallace. 1987. Experience and brain development. *Child Development* 58:539-559.

32. M. C. Diamond. 1988. The significance of enrichment. In *Enriching Heredity.* New York: The Free Press.

33. Hubel D. H. and T. N. Wiesel. 1970. The period of susceptibility to the physiological effects of unilateral eye closure in kittens. *Journal of Physiology* (London) 206: 419-436.

34. Kraemer, G. W. 1992. A psychobiological theory of attachment. *Behavioral and Brain Sciences* 15(3):502.

35. For recent syntheses of the literature on child abuse and neglect, see: United States Advisory Board on Child Abuse and Neglect. 1995. *A Nation's Shame: Fatal Child Abuse and Neglect in the United States.* Fifth Report. Washington; Trocme, N. and Caunce, C. 1995. The educational needs of abused and neglected children: A review of the literature. *Early Child Development and Care* 106(February):101-35.
For syntheses of the literature on the impact of poverty, see Huston, A. C. et. al. 1994. *Children and Poverty: Issues in Contemporary Research.* Special issue of *Child Development*, 65(2):275-282;
Renchler, R. 1993. Poverty and learning. *ERIC Digest.* Eugene, OR: ERIC Clearinghouse on Educational Management;
Sherman, A. 1994. *Wasting America's Future: The Children's Defense Fund Report on the Costs of Child Poverty.* Boston: Beacon Press.

36. Kestenbaum, R., E. A. Farber, L. A. Sroufe. 1989. Individual differences in empathy among preschoolers: Relation to attachment history. In N. Eisenberg, ed. *Empathy and Related Emotional Responses. New Directions for Child Development*, No. 44. San Francisco: Jossey-Bass (summer);
Sroufe, L. A. 1989. Infant-caregiver attachment and patterns of adaptation in preschool: The roots of maladaptation and competence. In M. Perlmutter, ed. *Minnesota Symposium in Child Psychology* 16:41-83. Hillsdale, NJ: Lawrence Erlbaum Associates.
Sroufe, L. A., E. Schork, F. Motti, N. Lawroski, and P. LaFreniere. 1984. The role of affect in social competence. In C. Izard, J. Kagan and R. Zajonc, eds. *Emotion, Cognition, and Behavior.* New York: Plenum.

37. Perry, Bruce D. 1996. Incubated in terror: Neurodevelopmental factors in the "cycle of violence." In J. D. Osofsky, ed. *Children, Youth and Violence: Searching for Solutions.* New York: Guilford Press.

38. Renken, B., B. Egeland, D. Marvinney, S. Mangelsdorf, and L. A. Sroufe. 1989. Early childhood antecedents of aggression and passive-withdrawal in early elementary school. *Journal of Personality* 57 (2):257-81;
Egeland, B. 1996. Mediators of the effects of child maltreatment on developmental adaptation in adolescence. In D. Cicchetti and S. L. Toth, eds. *The Effects of Trauma on the Developmental Process.* Rochester Symposium on Developmental Psychopathology, Vol. 8. Rochester: University of Rochester Press;
Sroufe, L. A. Psychopathology as development (in press). *Psychopathology.*

39. Greenspan, S. I. with B. L. Benderly. 1997. *The Growth of the Mind and the Endangered Origins of Intelligence.* Reading, MA: Addison Wesley.

40. Dawson, G., D. Hessl, and K. Frey. 1994. Social influences on early developing biological and behavioral systems related to risk for affective disorder. In *Development and Psychopathology.* Cambridge: Cambridge University Press, pp. 759-779.

41. Young, K. T., K. Davis, and C. Schoen. 1996. *The Commonwealth Fund Survey of Parents with Young Children.* New York: The Commonwealth Fund.

42. Ounce of Prevention Fund. 1996. *Starting Smart: How Early Experiences Affect Brain Development.* Chicago: Ounce of Prevention Fund, p. 5.

43. M. M. Cartwright and S. M. Smith. 1995. Increased cell death and reduced neural crest cell numbers in ethanol-exposed embryos: Partial basis for the fetal alcohol syndrome phenotype. *Alcohol: Clinical Experience and Research* 19 (April):378-38

44. Diamond, M. C. 1988. The significance of enrichment. In *Enriching Heredity.* New York: The Free Press.

45. Janzen, L. A., J. L. Nanson, and G. W. Block. 1995. Neuropsychological evaluation of preschoolers with FAS. *Neurotoxicol Teratol* 17 (May-June):273-279.

46. Wakschlag, L. S., B. B. Lahey, R. Loeber, S. M. Green, R. A. Gordon, and B. L. Leventhal. 1997. Maternal smoking during pregnancy and the risk of conduct disorder in boys; Archives of General Psychiatry; U. S. National Center for Health Statistics. 1996. *The Monthly Vital Statistics Reports.* Washington, DC: The Bureau of the Census.

47. Wakschlag, L. S., B. B. Lahey, R. Loeber, S. M. Green, R. A. Gordon, and B. L. Leventhal (in press). Maternal smoking during pregnancy and the risk of conduct disorder in boys. *Archives of General Psychiatry.*

48. Wakschlag, L. S., B. B. Lahey, R. Loeber, S. M. Green, R. A. Gordon, and B. L. Leventhal (in press). Maternal smoking during pregnancy and the risk of conduct disorder in boys. *Archives of General Psychiatry.*

49. Mayes, L. C. 1996. Early experience and the developing brain: The model of prenatal cocaine exposure. Presented at the conference: Brain Development in Young children: New Frontiers for Research, Policy, and Practice. The University of Chicago, June 13-14.

50. Mayes, L. C., M. H. Bornstein, K. Chawarska, and R. H. Granger. 1995. Information processing and developmental assessments in 3-month-old infants exposed prenatally to cocaine. *Pediatrics.* 95 (April): 539-545.

51. Spitz, R. A. 1945. Hospitalism: An inquiry into the genesis of psychiatric conditions in early childhood. Part I, *Psychoanalytic Study of the Child.* 1:53-74. See also:
Frank, D. A., P. E. Klass, F. Earls, and L. Eisenberg. 1996. Infants and young children in orphanages: One view from pediatrics and child psychiatry. *Pediatrics* 97 (April);

Carlson, M. and F. Earls (in press). Psychological and neuroendocrinological sequelae of early social deprivation in institutionalized children in Romania. In *Integrative Neurobiology of Affiliation*. New York: New York Academy of Science.

52. Goenjian, A. K., R. Yehuda, R. Pynoos et. al. 1996. Basal cortisol, dexamethasone suppression of cortisol, and MHPG in adolescents after the 1988 earthquake in Armenia. *American Journal of Psychiatry*. 153:929-934.

53. Frank, D. A., P. E. Klass, F. Earls, and L. Eisenberg. 1996. Infants and young children in orphanages: One view from pediatrics and child psychiatry. *Pediatrics* 97 (4)573.

54. Earlier studies of these children found that those adopted in the first six months of life show no deficits at any age tested; those adopted later continue to show deficits after adoption, although they improve dramatically. See Rutter, M. 1989. Age as an ambiguous variable in developmental research: Some epidemiological considerations from developmental psychopathology. *International Journal of Behavioral Development* 12(1)1-34.

55. Gunnar has conducted research examining cortisol levels of children attending child care programs in the U. S.

56. National Center for Children in Poverty. 1996. *One in Four: America's Youngest Poor*. New York: Columbia University.

57. Ramey, C. T. and S. Landesman Ramey. 1996. Prevention of intellectual disabilities: Early interventions to improve cognitive development. Birmingham: University of Alabama Civitan International Research Center.

58. Egeland, B., E. Carlson, and L. A. Sroufe. 1993. Resilience as process. In *Development and Psychopathology*. New York: Cambridge University Press, p. 520.

59. Erickson, M. F., J. Korfmacher, and B. Egeland. 1992. Attachments past and present: Implications for therapeutic intervention with mother-infant dyads. In *Development and Psychopathology*. New York: Cambridge University Press, pp. 495-507.

60. Als, H. and L. Gilkerson. 1995. Developmentally supportive care in the neonatal intensive care unit. *Zero to Three* (June/July):2-9.

61. Greenspan, S. I. 1997. *The Growth of the Mind and the Endangered Origins of Intelligence*. Reading, MA: Addison Wesley;
Greenspan, S. I. and S. Wider. 1997. *Facilitating Intellectual and Emotional Growth in Children With Special Needs*. Reading, MA: Addison Wesley; Greenspan, S. I. 1992. *Infancy and Early Childhood: The Practice of Clinical Assessment and Intervention with Emotional and Developmental Challenges*. Madison, CT: International Universities Press.

62. Rutter, M. 1996. Autism research: Prospects and priorities. *Journal of Autism and Developmental Disorders* 26(2, April):257-275.

63. Benasich, A. A. and P. Tallal (in press). Auditory temporal processing thresholds, habituation, and recognition memory over the first year. In *Infant Behavior and Development*.

64. Greenspan, S. I. 1997. *The Growth of the Mind and the Endangered Origins of Intelligence*. Reading, MA: Addison Wesley.

65. Perry, B. D. 1996. Incubated in terror: Neurodevelopmental factors in the "cycle of violence." In J. D. Osovsky, ed. *Children, Youth and Violence: Searching for Solutions*. New York: Guilford Press, p. 7.

66. Kraemer, G. W. 1992. A psychobiological theory of attachment. *Behavioral and Brain Sciences* 15(3):502.

67. Pons, T., P. E. Garraghty, A. K. Ommaya, J. H. Kaas, E. Taub, and M. Mishkin. 1991. Massive corticol reorganization after sensory deafferentation in adult macaques. *Science* 252, 1857-1860.

68. Werner, E. E. and R. S. Smith. 1992. *Overcoming the Odds: High-Risk Children from Birth to Adulthood*. Ithaca: Cornell University Press;
Carnegie Task Force on Learning in the Primary Grades. 1996. *Years of Promise: A Comprehensive Learning Strategy for America's Children*. New York: Carnegie Corporation;
Weissbourd, R. 1996. *The Vulnerable Child: What Really Hurts America's Children and What We Can Do About It*. New York: Addison Wesley.

69. Carnegie Task Force on Meeting the Needs of Young Children. 1994. *Starting Points: Meeting The Needs of Our Youngest Children*. New York: Carnegie Corporation of New York;
Children's Defense Fund. 1992. *The State of America's Children*. 1992. Washington, DC;
National Commission on Children. 1991. *Beyond Rhetoric: An New American Agenda for Children and Families*. Washington, DC;
National Health/Education Consortium. 1991. *Healthy Brain Development*. Report of a conference held in Baltimore, MD, December 6, 1990. Washington, DC: Institute for Educational Leadership and National Commission to Prevent Infant Mortality.

70. Galinsky, E., C. Howes, and S. Kontos. 1995. *The Family Care Training Study: Highlights of Findings*. New York: Families and Work Institute.

71. Dombro, A. L., N. Sazer O'Donnell, E. Galinsky, S. Gilkeson Melcher, and A. Farber. 1996. *Community Mobilization: Strategies to Support Young Children and Their Families*. New York: Families and Work Institute.

Sources for Sidebars

An Organ of Minor Importance

Aristotle. 1937 translation. *De Animalium Motu.* Trans. A.I. Peck, Cambridge: Harvard University Press. (Cited in Cerf, C. and V. Navasky. 1984. *The Experts Speak: The Definitive Compendium of Authoritative Misinformation.* New York: Pantheon);

Fallows, James. 1989. *More Like Us: Making America Great Again.* Boston: Houghton Mifflin.

The Neuroscientist's Toolbox

On PET scans: Chugani, H.T. Neuroimaging of developmental non-linearity and developmental pathologies. In R.W. Thatcher, G.R. Lyon, J. Rumsey, and N. Krasnegor, eds. *Developmental Neuroimaging: Mapping the development of brain and behavior.* San Diego: Academic Press.

On MRI and functional MRI: LeBihan, D. 1996. Functional MRI of the brain: Principles, applications, and limitations. *Journal of Neuroradiology,* Vol. 23, June 1996.

On EEG: Dawson, G. and K.W. Fischer. 1994. *Human Behavior and the Developing Brain.* New York: Guilford Press.

On cortisol analysis: Gunnar, M.R. 1996. Quality of care and the buffering of tress physiology: Its potential in protecting the developing human brain. University of Minnesota Institute of Child Development.

On the use of parents' videotapes. Bristol, M. 1996. Remarks at conference, Brain Development in Young Children: New Frontiers for Research, Policy, and Practice. University of Chicago, June 13-14.

The Quiet Crisis

Carnegie Task Force on Meeting the Needs of Young Children. 1994. *Starting Points: Meeting the Needs of Our Youngest Children.* New York, NY: Carnegie Corporation of New York.

On child abuse and neglect: National Center on Child Abuse and Neglect. 1996. *National Incidence Study of Child Abuse and Neglect* (Third annual study). Washington, DC: U. S. Department of Health and Human Services.

On low birthweight, teen pregnancy, prenatal care, and smoking during pregnancy: National Center for Health Statistics. 1996. *Health, United States, 1995* Hyattsville, MD: Public Health Service.

On uninsured children: 1995 data provided by Paul Fronstin, Employee Benefit Research Institute, Washington, DC.

On teen pregnancy: Department of Health and Human Services Press Office. 1997. Press release: Secretary Shalala launches national strategy to prevent teen pregnancy; New state-by-state data show declines in teen birth rates. Washington, DC (January 6).

On prenatal care: National Center for Chronic Disease Prevention and Health Promotion. 1995. *Maternal and Child Health.* Atlanta: National Centers for Disease Control and Prevention.

On immunization: Center for Disease Control. 1996. *National Immunization Survey.* Atlanta.

On boarder babies: U.S. Department of Health and Human Services, Office of Human Development Services Administration for Children, Youth, and Families Children's Bureau. 1994. *Report to the Congress: National Estimates on the Number of Boarder Babies, the Cost of Their Care, and the Number of Abandoned Infants.* Washington, DC: U.S. Department of Health and Human Services.

Following Children Through the Decades

Renken, B., B. Egeland, D. Marvinney, S. Mangelsdorf, and L.A. Sroufe, 1989. Early childhood antecedents of aggression and passive-withdrawal in early elementary school. *Journal of Personality,* 57(2, June).

Sroufe, L.A. and B. Egeland. 1991. Illustrations of person-environment interaction from a longitudinal study. In T. Wachs and R. Plomin, eds. *Conceptualization and Measurement of Organism-environment Interaction.* Washington D.C.: American Psychological Association.

Sroufe, L.A., B. Egeland, and T. Kreutzer. 1990. The fate of early experience following developmental change: Longitudinal approaches to individual adaptation in childhood. *Child Development.* 61:1363-1373.

Teo, A., E. Carlson, P.J. Mathieu, B. Egeland, and L.A. Sroufe. 1996. A prospective longitudinal study of psychosocial predictors of achievement. *Journal of School Psychology* 34 (3):285-306.

The Ecological Brain: An Anthropologist's View

Shore, B. 1996. *Culture in Mind: Cognition, Culture, and the Problem of Meaning.* New York: Oxford University Press.

Day-to-Day Care of Young Children's Brains

Carnegie Task Force on Meeting the Needs of Young Children. 1994. *Starting Points: Meeting the Needs of Our Youngest Children: The Report of the Carnegie Task Force on Meeting the Needs of Young Children.* New York, NY: Carnegie Corporation of New York.

Materials prepared for the *I Am Your Child* Public Engagement Campaign.

Gauging Attachment

Erickson, M.F., J. Korfmacher, and B. Egeland, Attachments past and present: Implications for therapeutic intervention with mother-infant dyads." In *Development and Psychopathology.* New York: Cambridge University Press, 1992, pp. 495-507.

Droege, K.L. 1996. The forgotten social development goal in Head Start. *Jobs & Capital.* 5(spring), feature article 4.

Galinsky, E., C. Howes, S. Kontos, and M. Shinn. 1994. *The Study of Children in Family Child Care and Relative Care.* New York: Families and Work Institute.

Gunnar, M.R. 1996. Quality of care and the buffering of stress physiology: Its potential role in protecting the developing human brain. University of Minnesota: Institute of Child Development.

Howes, C. and C.E. Hamilton. 1993. Child care for young children. In B. Spodek, ed. *Handbook of Research on the Education of Young Children.* New York: Macmillan, pp. 322-336.

Lieberman, A. F. and C.H. Zeanah. 1995. Disorders of attachment in infancy. *Infant Psychiatry 4 (3):*571-587.

Kraemer, G.W. 1992. A psychobiological theory of attachment. *Behavioral and Brain Sciences,* Vol. 15, No. 3, 1992, pp. 493-511.

Waters, E and K. Deane. 1985. Defining and assessing individual differences in attachment relationships: Q-methodology and the organization of behavior in infancy and early childhood. *Monographs of the Society for Research in Child Development.* 50(a, Serial No. 209):41-65.

Prevention and Early Intervention

Barnett, W.S. 1995. Long-term effects of early childhood programs on cognitive and school outcomes. *The Future of Children: Long-Term Outcomes of Early Childhood Programs* 5 (3):25-50.

Campbell, F.A. and C.T. Ramey. 1994. Effects of early intervention on intellectual and academic achievement: A follow-up study of children from low-income families. *Child Development* 65:684-698.

McCarton, C.M., F.C. Bennett, M.C. McCormick, and Curtis L. Meinen. 1977. Results at age 8 years of early intervention for low-birth-weight premature infants. *Journal of the American Medical Association* 277 (January 8):126-32.

Olds, D. 1977. Primary prevention works. In G. Albee and T. Gullotta, eds. *Issues in Children's and Families Lives* Vol. 6. CA:Sage Publications.

Shore, R. *1996. Family Support and Parent Education: Opportunities for Scaling Up.* New York, NY: Carnegie Corporation of New York.

Yoshikawa, H. 1995. Long-term effects of early childhood programs on social outcomes and delinquency. *The Future of Children: Long-Term Outcomes of Early Childhood Programs* 5 (3):51-75.

Who is a Caregiver? Child Care and Early Education

Bureau of Labor Statistics. 1995. Marital and family characteristics of workers. In *Special Labor Force Report* 64(March). Washington, DC: Bureau of Labor Statistics.

Bureau of Labor Statistics. 1995. *Handbook of Labor Statistics.* Bulletin 2340. Washington, DC: Bureau of Labor Statistics.

Carnegie Task Force on Learning in the Primary Grades. *Years of Promise: A Comprehensive Learning Strategy for America's Children.* New York, NY: Carnegie Corporation of New York.

Cost, Quality, and Child Outcomes Study Team. 1995. *Cost, Quality, and Child Outcomes in Child Care Centers.* Denver, CO: Department of Economics, University of Colorado at Denver.

Galinsky, E., Bond, J.T., and Friedman, D.E. 1993. *The Changing Workforce: Highlights of the National Study.* New York, NY: Families and Work Institute.

Galinsky, E. and D.E. Friedman. 1993. *Education Before School: Investing in Quality Child Care.* Commissioned by the Committee for Economic Development. New York, NY: Scholastic, Inc.

Galinsky, E., C. Howes, S. Kontos, and M. Shinn. 1994. *The Study of Children in Family Child Care and Relative Care.* New York: Families and Work Institute.

Hofferth, S.L., A. Brayfield, S. Deich, and P. Holcomb 1991. *National Child Care Survey, 1990.* Washington, DC: The Urban Institute.

Howes, C., E. Smith, and E. Galinsky. 1994. *The Florida Child Care Quality Improvement Study: Interim Report.* New York, NY: Families and Work Institute.

Kagan, S.L. and N.E. Cohen. 1997. *Solving the Quality Problem : A Vision for America's Early Care and Education System.* New Haven: Yale Bush Center.

Kisker, E.E., S.L. Hofferth, D.A. Phillips, and E. Farquhar. 1991. *A Profile of Child Care Settings, Early Education and Care in 1990.* Vol 1. Princeton, NJ: Mathematica Policy Research, Inc.

Kontos, S., C. Howes, M. Shinn, and E. Galinsky. 1994. *Quality in Family Child Care and Relative Care.* New York: Teachers College Press.

Morgan, G., S.L. Azer, J.B. Costley, A. Genser, I.F. Goodman, J. Lombardi, J. and B. McGimsey. 1993. *Making a Career of It: The State of the States Report on Career Development in Early Care and Education.* Boston, MA: Wheelock College, The Center for Career Development in Early Care and Education.

Phillips, D.A., D. Mekos, S. Scarr, K. McCartney And M. Abbott-Shim (in press). *Paths to Quality in Child Care: Structural and Contextual Influences on Children's Classroom Environments.* Charlottesville, VA: University of Virginia.

Whitebook, M., C. Howes, and D.A. Phillips. 1990. *Who Cares? Child Care Teachers and the Quality of Care in America.* Final report of the National Child Care Staffing Study. Oakland, CA: Child Care Employee Project.

Whitebook, M., D. A. Phillips, and C. Howes. 1993. *National Child Care Starring Study Revisited: Four Years in the Life of Center-Based Child Care.* Oakland, CA: Child Care Employee Project.

Willer, B., S.L. Hofferth, E.E. Kisker, P. Divine-Hawkin., E. Farquhar, and F.B. Glanz. 1991. *The Demand and Supply of Child Care in 1990.* Washington, DC: National Association for the Education of Young Children.

Tough Questions

Families and Work Institute. 1995. *Women: The New Providers.* New York: Families and Work Institute.

Frank, D.A., P.E. Klass, F Earls, and L. Eisenberg. 1996. Infants and young children in orphanages: One view from pediatrics and child psychiatry. *Pediatrics* 97 (April).

Bibliography

Allen, M., P. Brown, and B. Finlay. 1992. *Helping Children by Strengthening Families: A Look at Family Support Programs.* Washington, DC: Children's Defense Fund.

Als, H. and L. Gilkerson. 1995. Developmentally supportive care in the neonatal intensive care unit. *Zero to Three* (June/July):2-9.

Als, H., G. Lawhon, F. H. Duffy, G. B. McAnulty, R. Gibes-Grossman, and J. G. Blickman. 1994. Individualized developmental care for the very low-birth-weight preterm infant: Medical and neurofunctional effects. *Journal of the American Medical Association* 272 (September 21):853-891.

Angleitner, A. and J. Strelau, eds. 1994. *Explorations in Temperament: International Perspectives on Theory and Measurement.* New York: Plenum.

Archives of General Psychiatry; U. S. National Center for Health Statistics. 1996. *The Monthly Vital Statistics Reports.* Washington, DC: The Bureau of the Census.

Barnett, W. S. 1993. New wine in old bottles: Increasing the coherence of early childhood care and education policy. *Early Childhood Research Quarterly* 8:519-558.

Barnett, W. S. 1995. Long term effects of early childhood programs on cognitive and school outcomes. *The Future of Children: Long-Term Outcomes of Early Childhood Programs* 5 (3):25-50.

Benasich, A. A. and P. Tallal (in press). Auditory temporal processing thresholds, habituation, and recognition memory over the first year. In *Infant Behavior and Development.*

Black, J. E. and Greenough, W. T. 1986. Induction of pattern in neural structure by experience: Implications for cognitive development. In M. E. Lamb, A. L. Brown, and B. Rogoff, eds. *Advances in Developmental Psychology.* Vol. 4. Hillsdale, NJ: Lawrence Earlbaum Assoc., pp. 1-50.

Boyer, E. L. 1991. *Ready to Learn: A Mandate for the Nation.* Princeton: Carnegie Foundation for the Advancement of Teaching.

Bristol, M. M., D. J. Cohen, E. J. Costello, M. Denckla, T. J. Eckberg, R. Kallen, H. C. Kraemer, C. Lord, R. Maurer, W. J. McIlvane, N. Minshew, M. Sigman, and M. A. Spence. 1996. State of the science in autism: A view from the National Institutes of Health. *Journal of Autism and Developmental Disorders* 26 (2):121-154.

Brooks-Gunn, J., F. Liaw, and P. K. Klebanov. 1992. Effects of early intervention on cognitive function of low birth weight preterm infants. *The Journal of Pediatrics* 120 (March):350-358.

Brooks-Gunn, J., M. C. McCormick, S. Shapiro, A. A. Benasich, and G. W. Black. 1994. The effects of early education intervention on maternal employment, public assistance, and health insurance: The Infant Health and Development Program. *American Journal of Public Health* 84 (June):924-930.

Bureau of Labor Statistics. 1965. Marital and family characteristics of workers. In *Special Labor Force Report* 64(March). Washington, DC: Bureau of Labor Statistics.

Bureau of Labor Statistics. 1995. *Handbook of Labor Statistics.* Bulletin 2340. Washington, DC: Bureau of Labor Statistics.

Campbell, F. A. and C. T. Ramey. 1994. Effects of early intervention on intellectual and academic achievement: A follow-up study of children from low-income families. *Child Development* 65:684-698.

Campbell, F. A. and C. T. Ramey. 1995. Cognitive and school outcomes for high-risk African-American students at middle adolescence: Positive effects of early intervention. *American Educational Research Journal* 32(4):743-772.

Carlson, M. and F. Earls (in press). Psychological and neuroendocrinological sequelae of early social deprivation in institutionalized children in Romania. In *Integrative Neurobiology of Affiliation.* New York: New York Academy of Science.

Carnegie Task Force on Learning in the Primary Grades. 1996. *Years of Promise: A Comprehensive Learning Strategy for America's Children.* New York: Carnegie Corporation of New York.

Carnegie Task Force on Meeting the Needs of Young Children. 1994. *Starting Points: Meeting the Needs of Our Youngest Children.* New York: Carnegie Corporation of New York.

Cartwright, M. M. and S. M. Smith. 1995. Increased cell death and reduced neural crest cell numbers in ethanol-exposed embryos: Partial basis for the fetal alcohol syndrome phenotype. *Alcohol: Clinical Experience and Research* 19 (April):378-386.

Centers for Disease Control. 1996. *National Immunization Survey.* Atlanta: Centers for Disease Control.

Cerf, C. and V. Navasky. 1984. *The Experts Speak: The Definitive Compendium of Authoritative Misinformation.* New York: Pantheon.

Chugani, H. T. 1997. Neuroimaging of developmental non-linearity and developmental pathologies. In R. W. Thatcher, G. R. Lyon, J. Rumsey, and N. Krasnegor, eds. *Developmental Neuroimaging: Mapping the Development of Brain and Behavior.* San Diego: Academic Press.

Cost, Quality, and Child Outcomes Study Team. 1995. *Cost, Quality, and Child Outcomes in Child Care Centers.* Denver, CO: Department of Economics, University of Colorado at Denver.

Curtiss, S. 1981. Feral children. In J. Wortis, ed. *Mental Retardation and Developmental Disabilities* XII. New York: Brunner/Mazel.

Dawson, G. and K. W. Fischer. 1994. *Human Behavior and the Developing Brain.* New York: Guilford Press.

Dawson, G., D. Hessl, and K. Frey. 1994. Social influences on early developing biological and behavioral systems related to risk for affective disorder. In *Development and Psychopathology.* Cambridge: Cambridge University Press, pp. 759-779.

Diamond, M. C. 1988. The significance of enrichment. In *Enriching Heredity.* New York: The Free Press.

Dombro, A. L., N. Sazer O'Donnell, E. Galinsky, S. Gilkeson Melcher, and A. Farber. 1996. *Community Mobilization: Strategies to Support Young Children and Their Families.* New York: Families and Work Institute.

Droege, K. L. 1996. The forgotten social development goal in Head Start. *Jobs and Capital* 5(Spring), feature article 4.

Earls, F. and M. Carlson. 1994. Promoting human capability as an alternative to early crime prevention. In P-OH. Wikstrom, R. V. Clarke and J. McCord, eds. *Integrating Crime Prevention Strategies: Propensity and Opportunity.* Stockholm, Sweden: National Council on Crime Prevention, pp. 141-168.

Earls, F. and Maya Carlson. 1993. Towards sustainable development for American families. *Daedalus* 122:93-121.

Egeland, B., E. Carlson, and L. A. Sroufe. 1993. Resilience as process. In *Development and Psychopathology.* Cambridge: Cambridge University Press.

Erickson, M. F., J. Korfmacher, and B. Egeland. 1992. Attachments past and present: Implications for therapeutic intervention with mother-infant dyads. In *Development and Psychopathology.* New York: Cambridge University Press, pp. 495-507.

Fallows, J. 1989. *More Like Us: Making America Great Again.* Boston: Houghton Mifflin Co.

Families and Work Institute. 1995. *Women: The New Providers.* New York: Families and Work Institute.

Frank, D. A., P. E. Klass, F. Earls, and L. Eisenberg. 1996. Infants and young children in orphanages: One view from pediatrics and child psychiatry. *Pediatrics* 97 (April).

Galinsky, E. and D. E. Friedman. 1993. *Education Before School: Investing in Quality Child Care.* Commissioned by the Committee for Economic Development. New York: Scholastic, Inc.

Galinsky, E. and J. David. 1988. *The Preschool Years: Family Strategies That Work From Experts and Parents.* New York: Ballantine Books.

Galinsky, E., C. Howes, and S. Kontos. 1995. *The Family Child Care Training Study: Highlights of Findings.* New York: Families and Work Institute.

Galinsky, E., C. Howes, S. Kontos, and M. Shinn. 1994. *The Study of Children in Family Child Care and Relative Care: Highlights of Findings.* New York: Families and Work Institute.

Galinsky, E., J. T. Bond, and D. E. Friedman. 1993. *The Changing Workforce: Highlights of the National Study.* New York: Families and Work Institute.

Goenjian, A. K., R. Yehuda, R. Pynoos, A. M. Steinberg, M. Tashijian, R. Kwei Yang, L. M. Najarian, and L. A. Fairbanks. 1996. Basal cortisol, dexamethasone suppression of cortisol, and MHPG in adolescents after the 1988 earthquake in Armenia. *American Journal of Psychiatry* 153 (7):929-934.

Gomby, D. S., M. B. Larner, C. S. Stevenson, E. M. Lewit, and R. E. Behrman. 1995. Long-term outcomes of early childhood programs: Analysis and recommendations. *The Future of Children* 5(3).

Greenough, W. T., J. E. Black, and C. Wallace. 1987. Experience and brain development. *Child Development* 58:539-559.

Greenough, W. T., T. A. Comery and R. Shah. 1995. Differential rearing alters spine density on medium-sized spiny neurons in the rat corpus striatum: Evidence for association of morphological plasticity with early response gene expression. *Neurobiology of Learning and Memory* 63:217-219.

Greenspan, S. I. 1992. *Infancy and Early Childhood: The Practice of Clinical Assessment and Intervention with Emotional and Developmental Challenges.* Madison, CT: International Universities Press.

Greenspan, S. I. and S. Wider. 1997. *Facilitating Intellectual and Emotional Growth in Children With Special Needs.* Reading, MA: Addison Wesley.

Greenspan, S. I. with J. Salmon. 1994. *The Challenging Child: Understanding, Raising, and Enjoying the Five "Difficult" Types of Children.* Reading, MA: Addison Wesley.

Greenspan, S. I., with B. L. Benderly. 1997. *The Growth of the Mind and the Endangered Origins of Intelligence.* Reading, MA: Addison Wesley.

Gunnar, M. R. 1996. Quality of care and the buffering of stress physiology: Its potential in protecting the developing human brain. University of Minnesota Institute of Child Development.

Halverson, C. F. Jr., G. A. Kohnstamm, R. P. Martin, eds. 1994. *The Developing Structure of Temperament and Personality from Infancy to Adulthood.* Hillsdale, NJ: Lawrence Erlbaum Associates.

Hanson, R. A. 1992. Prescription for literacy: Providing critical educational experiences. *ERIC Digest.* Bloomington: ERIC Clearinghouse on Reading and Communication Skills.

Harris, I. B. May 31, 1996. Helen Harris Perlman Lecture. "New knowledge about the human brain and its meaning for early childhood development."

Hofer, M. A. 1988. On the nature and function of prenatal behavior. In W. Smotherman and S. Robinson, eds. *Behavior of the Fetus.* Caldwell, NJ: Telford Press.

Hofer, M. A. 1995. Hidden regulators: Implications for a new understanding of attachment, separation, and loss. In S. Goldberg, R. Muir and J. Kerr, eds. *Attachment Theory: Social Developmental and Clinical Perspectives.* Hillsdale, NJ: The Analytic Press.

Hofferth, S. L., A. Brayfield, S. Deich, and P. Holcomb. 1991. *National Child Care Survey* 1990. Washington, DC: The Urban Institute.

Howes, C. 1990. Can the age of entry into child care and the quality of child care predict adjustment in kindergarten? *Developmental Psychology* 26: 292-303.

Howes, C. and C. E. Hamilton. 1993. Child care for young children. In Bernard Spodek, ed. *Handbook of Research on the Education of Young Children.* New York: Macmillan, pp. 322-336.

Howes, C., E. Smith, and E. Galinsky. 1994. *The Florida Child Care Quality Improvement Study: Interim Report.* New York: Families and Work Institute.

Huston, A. C. et al. 1994. Children and poverty: Issues in contemporary research. Special issue of *Child Development* 65(2):275-82.

Huston, A. C., ed. 1991. *Children in Poverty: Child Development and Public Policy.* New York: Cambridge University Press.

Huttenlocher, P. R. 1984. Synapse elimination and plasticity in developing human cerebral cortex. *American Journal of Mental Deficiency* 88:488-496.

Infant Health and Development Program. 1990. Enhancing the outcomes of low-birth-weight, premature infants: A multisite, randomized trial. *Journal of the American Medical Association* 263 (22):3035-3041.

Jabs, C. 1996. Your baby's brain. *Working Mother* (November):24-28.

Janzen, L. A., J. L. Nanson, and G. W. Block. 1995. Neuropsychological evaluation of preschoolers with FAS. *Neurotoxicol Teratol 17* (May-June):273-279.

Kagan, S. L. and N. E. Cohen. (1997). *Solving the Quality Problem: A Vision for America's Early Care and Education System.* New Haven: Yale University.

Kempermann,G., H.G. Kuhn, and F.H. Gage. 1997 More hippocampal neurons in adult mice living in an enriched environment. *Nature* 386 (April 3):493-95.

Kestenbaum, R., E. A. Farber, L. A. Sroufe. 1989. Individual differences in empathy among preschoolers: Relation to attachment history. In N. Eisenberg, ed. Empathy and Related Emotional Responses. *New Directions for Child Development* 44 (Summer). San Francisco: Jossey-Bass.

Kisker, E. E., S. L. Hofferth, D. A. Phillips, and E. Farquhar. 1991. *A Profile of Child Care Settings, Early Education and Care in 1990.* Vol. 1. Princeton, NJ: Mathematica Policy Research, Inc.

Kontos, S., C. Howes, M. Shinn, and E. Galinsky. 1994. *Quality in Family Child Care and Relative Care.* New York: Teachers College Press.

Kotulak, R. 1996. *Inside the Brain: Revolutionary Discoveries of How the Mind Works.* Kansas City, MO: Andrews and McMeel.

Kraemer, G. W. 1992. A psychobiological theory of attachment. *Behavioral and Brain Sciences* 15 (3):493-511.

L. A. Sroufe, B. Egeland, and T. Kreutzer. 1990. The fate of early experience following developmental change: Longitudinal approaches to individual adaptation in childhood. *Child Development* 61:1363-1373.

Le Bihan, D. 1996. Functional MRI of the brain: Principles, applications and limitations. *Journal of Neuroradiology* 23 (June).

Lieberman, A. F. and C. H. Zeanah. 1995. Disorders of attachment in infancy. *Infant Psychiatry* 4 (3):571-587.

Lock, J. L. 1993. *The Child's Path to Spoken Language.* Cambridge: Harvard University Press.

Martin, R. P. 1994. Child temperament and common problems in schooling: Hypotheses about causal connections. *Journal of School Psychology* 32:119-134.

Mayes, L. C., M. H. Bornstein, K. Chawarska, and R. H. Granger. 1995. Information processing and developmental assessments in 3-month-old infants exposed prenatally to cocaine. *Pediatrics* 95 (4):539-545.

Mayes, L. C., M. H. Bornstein, K. Chawarska, O. M. Haynes, and R. H. Granger. 1996. Impaired regulation of arousal in 3-month-old infants exposed prenatally to cocaine and other drugs. In *Development and Psychopathology.* Cambridge: Cambridge University Press, pp. 29-42.

McCarton, C. M., F. C. Bennett, M. C. McCormick, and C. L. Meinen. 1977. Results at age 8 years of early intervention for low-birth-weight premature infants. *Journal of the American Medical Association* 277 (January 8, 1977):126-32.

Morgan, G., S. L. Azer, J. B. Costley, A. Genser, I. F. Goodman, J. Lombardi, and B. McGimsey. 1993. *Making a Career of It: The State of the States Report on Career Development in Early Care and Education.* Boston: Wheelock College, The Center for Career Development in Early Care and Education.

National Center for Children in Poverty. 1996. *One in Four: America's Youngest Poor.* New York: Columbia University.

National Center on Child Abuse and Neglect. 1996. *National Incidence Study of Child Abuse and Neglect* (Third annual study). Washington, DC: Department of Health and Human Services.

National Center for Chronic Disease Prevention and Health Promotion. 1995. *Maternal and Child Health*. Atlanta: Centers for Disease Control.

National Commission on Children. 1991. *Beyond Rhetoric: A New American Agenda for Children and Families*. Washington, DC: National Commission on Children.

National Center for Health Statistics. 1996. *Health, United States, 1995* Hyattsville, MD: Public Health Service.

National Health/Education Consortium. 1991. *Healthy Brain Development*. Report of a conference held in Baltimore, MD, December 6, 1990. Washington, DC: Institute for Educational Leadership and National Commission to Prevent Infant Mortality.

Olds, D. 1997. The prenatal/early infancy project: Fifteen years later. In G. W. Albee and T. P. Gullotta, eds. *Primary Prevention Works*, Vol. VI of *Issues in Children and Families Lives*. Thousand Oaks, CA: Sage Publications, pp. 41-67.

Ounce of Prevention Fund. 1996. *Starting Smart: How Early Experiences Affect Brain Development*. Chicago: Ounce of Prevention Fund.

Perry, B. D. 1993. Neurodevelopment and the neurophysiology of trauma I: Conceptional considerations for clinical work with maltreated children. *The Advisor* 6 (Spring 1993):1.

Perry, B. D. 1993. Neurodevelopment and the neurophysiology of trauma II: Clinical work along the alarm-rear-terror continuum. *The Advisor* 6 (Summer 1993):1.

Perry, B. D. 1994. Neurobiological sequelae of childhood trauma: PTSD in children. In M. Murberg, ed. *Catecholamine Function in PTSD*. Washington, DC: American Psychiatric Press.

Perry, B. D. 1996. Incubated in terror: Neurodevelopmental factors in the "cycle of violence." In J. D. Osovsky, ed. *Children, Youth and Violence: Searching for Solutions*. New York: Guilford Press.

Perry, B. D., R. A. Pollard, T. L. Blakley, W. L. Baker, and D. Vigilante. 1995. Childhood trauma, the neurobiology of adaptation, and "use-dependent" development of the brain: How "states" become "traits". *Infant Mental Health Journal* 259 (4):271-291.

Pfannenstiel, J., T. Lambson, V. Yarnell. 1991. *Second Wave Study of the Parents as Teachers Program*. St. Louis: Parents as Teachers National Center, Inc.

Pfannenstiel, J., T. Lambson, V. Yarnell. 1996. *The Parents as Teachers Program: Longitudinal Follow-Up to the Second Wave Study*. Oakland Pk, KS: Research and Training Associates, Inc.

Phillips, D. A., D. Mekos, S. Scarr, K. McCartney and M. Abbott-Shim (in press). *Paths to Quality in Child Care: Structural and Contextual Influences on Children's Classroom Environments*. Charlottesville, VA: University of Virginia.

Pons, T., P. E. Garraghty, A. K. Ommaya, J. H. Kaas, E. Taub, and M. Mishkin. 1991. Massive corticol reorganization after sensory deafferentation in adult macaques. *Science* 252: 1857-1860.

Prior, M. 1992. Childhood temperament. *Journal of Child Psychology and Psychiatry* 33:249-279.

Rakic, P. 1985. Limits of neurogenesis in primates. *Science* 227 (March 1):1054-1056.

Rakic, P. 1988. Specification of cerebral cortical areas. *Science* 241 (July 8):170-176.

Rakic, P. 1996. Development of the cerebral cortex in human and nonhuman primates. In M. Lewis, ed. *Child and Adolescent Psychiatry: A Comprehensive Textbook*, Second Edition. Williams and Wilkins, pp. 9-30.

Rakic, P., J. Bourgeois and P. S. Goldman-Rakic. 1994. Synaptic development of the cerebral cortex: Implications for learning, memory, and mental illness. In J. van Pelt, M. A. Corner, H. B. M. Uylings and P. H. Lopes da Silva, eds. *The Self-organizing Brain: From Growth Cones to Functional Networks*. Elsevier Science BV.

Ramey, C. T. and S. Landesman Ramey. 1992. At risk does not mean doomed. National Health/Education Consortium. *Occasional Paper #4* (June).

Ramey, C. T. and S. Landesman Ramey. 1996. Prevention of intellectual disabilities: Early interventions to improve cognitive development. Birmingham: University of Alabama Civitan International Research Center.

Ramey, C. T., D. M. Bryant, B. H. Wasik, J. J. Sparling, K. H. Fendt, and L. M. LaVange. 1992. Infant health and development program for low birth weight, premature infants: Program elements, family participation, and child intelligence. *Pediatrics* 3 (March):454-465.

Renchler, R. Poverty and learning. 1993. *ERIC Digest*. Eugene, Oregon: ERIC Clearinghouse on Educational Management.

Renken, B., B. Egeland, D. Marvinney, S. Mangelsdorf, and L. A. Sroufe. 1989. Early childhood antecedents of aggression and passive-withdrawal in early elementary school. *Journal of Personality* 57 (2):257-81.

Rossi, R. and A. Montgomery, eds. 1994. *Education Reforms and Students at Risk: A Review of the Current State of the Art*. Washington, DC: U. S. Education Department, American Institutes for Research.

Rutter, M. 1989. Age as an ambiguous variable in developmental research: Some epidemiological considerations from developmental psychopathology. *International Journal of Behavioral Development* 12(1)1-34.

Rutter, M. 1996. Autism research: Prospects and priorities. *Journal of Autism and Developmental Disorders* 26(2, April):257-275.

Schweinhart, L. J., H. V. Barnes, and D. P. Weikart. 1993. *Significant Benefits: The High/Scope Perry Preschool Study Through Age 27*. Monographs of the High/Scope Educational Research Foundation, No. 10. Ypsilanti, MI: High/Scope Press.

Shore, B. 1996. *Culture in Mind: Cognition, Culture, and the Problem of Meaning*. New York: Oxford University Press.

Shore, R. 1996. *Family Support and Parent Education: Opportunities for Scaling Up*. New York: Carnegie Corporation of New York.

Siegel, D. F. and R. A. Hanson. 1992. Prescription for literacy: Providing critical educational experiences. *ERIC Digest*. Bloomington: ERIC Clearinghouse on Reading and Communication Skills.

Spitz, R.A. 1945. Hospitalism: An inquiry into the genesis of psychiatric conditions in early childhood. Part I, *Psychoanalytic Study of the Child*. 1:53-74.

Sroufe, L. A. 1989. Infant-caregiver attachment and patterns of adaptation in preschool: The roots of maladaptation and competence. In M. Perlmutter, ed. *Minnesota Symposium in Child Psychology* 16:41-83. Hillsdale, NJ: Lawrence Erlbaum Associates.

Sroufe, L. A. and B. Egeland. 1991. Illustrations of person-environment interaction from a longitudinal study. In T. Wachs and R. Plomin, eds. *Conceptualization and Measurement of Organism-environment Interaction*. Washington, DC: American Psychological Association.

Sroufe, L. A. Psychopathology as development (in press). *Psychopathology*.

Sroufe, L. A., E. Schork, F. Motti, N. Lawroski, and P. LaFreniere. 1984. The role of affect in social competence. In C. Izard, J. Kagan and R. Zajonc, eds. *Emotion, Cognition, and Behavior*. New York: Plenum.

Teglasi, H. 1995. Assessment of temperament. *ERIC Digest*. Greensboro, NC: ERIC Clearinghouse on Counseling and Student Services.

Teo, A., E. Carlson, P. J. Mathieu, B. Egeland, and L. A. Sroufe. 1996. A prospective longitudinal study of psychosocial predictors of achievement. *Journal of School Psychology* 34 (3):285-306.

Trocme, N. and C. Caunce. 1995. The educational needs of abused and neglected children: A review of the literature. *Early Development and Care*. 106 (February): 101-35.

U. S. Department of Health and Human Services Press Office. 1997. Press release: Secretary Shalala launches national strategy to prevent teen pregnancy; New state-by-state data show declines in teen birth rates. Washington, DC (January 6).

U. S. National Center for Health Statistics. 1996. *The Monthly Vital Statistics Reports*. Washington, DC: The Bureau of the Census.

United States Advisory Board on Child Abuse and Neglect. 1995. *A Nation's Shame: Fatal Child Abuse and Neglect in the United States*. Fifth Report. Washington, Trocme, Nico; Caunce, Carrie 1995. The Educational Needs of Abused and Neglected Children: A Review of the Literature.

Viadero, D. 1996. Brain trust. *Education Week* XVI (September 18):1-2.

Wakschlag, L. S., B. B. Lahey, R. Loeber, S. M. Green, R. A. Gordon, and B. L. Leventhal. 1997. Maternal smoking during pregnancy and the risk of conduct disorder in boys. *Archives of General Psychiatry*.

Walker, T. B., G. G. Rodriguez, D. L. Johnson, and C. P. Cortez. 1995. Avance Parent-Child Education Program. In S. Smith and I. E. Sigel, eds. *Advances in Applied Developmental Psychology: Vol. 9. Two Generation Programs for Families in Poverty: A New Intervention Strategy*. Norwood, NJ: Ablex, pp. 67-90.

Waters, E. and K. Deane. 1985. Defining and assessing individual differences in attachment relationships: Q-methodology and the organization of behavior in infancy and early childhood. *Monographs of the Society for Research in Child Development* 50(1-2):41-65.

Weissbourd, R. 1996. *The Vulnerable Child: What Really Hurts America's Children and What We Can Do About It*. New York: Addison Wesley.

Werner, E. E. and R. S. Smith. 1992. *Overcoming the Odds: High-Risk Children from Birth to Adulthood*. Ithaca: Cornell University Press.

Whitebook, M., C. Howes, and D. A. Phillips. 1990. *Who Cares? Child Care Teachers and the Quality of Care in America*. Final report of the National Child Care Staffing Study. Oakland, CA: Child Care Employee Project.

Whitebook, M., D. A. Phillips, and C. Howes. 1993. *National Child Care Staffing Study Revisited: Four Years in the Life of Center-Based Child Care*. Oakland, CA: Child Care Employee Project.

Willer, B., S. L. Hofferth, E. E. Kisker, P. Divine-Hawkins, E. Farquhar, and F. B. Glanz. 1991. *The Demand and Supply of Child Care in 1990: Joint Findings from The National Child Care Survey 1990 and A Profile of Child Care Settings*. Washington, DC: National Association for the Education of Young Children.

Yoshikawa, H. 1995. Long–term effects of early childhood programs on social outcomes and delinquency. *The Future of Children: Long-Term Outcomes of Early Childhood Programs*. 5 (3): 51-75.

Young, K. T., K. Davis, and C. Schoen. 1996. *The Commonwealth Fund Survey of Parents with Young Children*. New York: The Commonwealth Fund.